BOURNE
D0314320

ALSO BY BOB HARPER

Are You Ready!

the
skinny
rules

Conversion Chart

Oven Temperatures:
130°C = 250°F = Gas mark ½
150°C = 300°F = Gas mark 2
180°C = 350°F = Gas mark 4
190°C = 375°F = Gas mark 5
200°C = 400°F = Gas mark 6
220°C = 425°F = Gas mark 7
230°C = 450°F = Gas mark 8

Spoon Measures:
1 level tablespoon flour = 15g
1 heaped tablespoon flour = 28g
1 level tablespoon sugar = 28g
1 level tablespoon butter = 15g

American solid measures
1 cup rice US = 225g
1 cup flour US = 115g
1 cup butter US = 225g
1 stick butter US = 115g
1 cup dried fruit US = 225g
1 cup brown sugar US = 180g
1 cup granulated sugar US = 225g

Liquid measures
1 cup US = 275ml
1 pint US = 550ml
1 quart US = 900ml

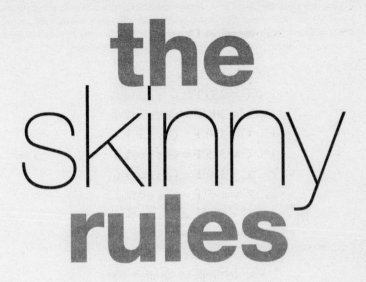

the skinny rules

BOB HARPER

with Greg Critser

BANTAM PRESS

LONDON • TORONTO • SYDNEY • AUCKLAND • JOHANNESBURG

No book can replace the diagnostic expertise and medical advice of a trusted physician. Please be certain to consult your doctor before making any decisions that affect your health or extreme changes in your diet, particularly if you suffer from any medical condition or have any symptom that may require attention.

TRANSWORLD PUBLISHERS
61–63 Uxbridge Road, London W5 5SA
A Random House Group Company
www.transworldbooks.co.uk

First published in Great Britain
in 2012 by Bantam Press
an imprint of Transworld Publishers

Copyright © Bob Harper, 2012

Bob Harper has asserted his right under the Copyright, Designs and Patents Act 1988 to be identified as the author of this work.

A CIP catalogue record for this book
is available from the British Library.

ISBN 9780593071618

This book is sold subject to the condition that it shall not, by way of trade or otherwise, be lent, resold, hired out, or otherwise circulated without the publisher's prior consent in any form of binding or cover other than that in which it is published and without a similar condition, including this condition, being imposed on the subsequent purchaser.

Addresses for Random House Group Ltd companies outside the UK
can be found at: www.randomhouse.co.uk
The Random House Group Ltd Reg. No. 954009

The Random House Group Limited supports the Forest Stewardship Council (FSC®), the leading international forest-certification organization. Our books carrying the FSC label are printed on FSC®-certified paper. FSC is the only forest-certification scheme endorsed by the leading environmental organizations, including Greenpeace. Our paper procurement policy can be found at www.randomhouse.co.uk/environment.

Typeset in 11/15 pt Minion
Printed and bound by
CPI Group (UK) Ltd, Croydon, CR0 4YY

2 4 6 8 10 9 7 5 3 1

CONTENTS

PART II:

THE SKINNY WAY

PART III:

THE SKINNY TOOLS

INTRODUCTION

Eat What I Tweet!

Sometimes big ideas come from small places.

From, say, a tweet.

That's how this book came about.

I was on my way back from a taping of *The Biggest Loser* when I got a phone call. It was from Ben, the husband of Olivia, who won Season 11.

"I'm following you," he told me. Pretty sure he didn't mean he was stalking me, I still had to ask what on earth he was talking about.

"I'm following what you eat—your meals you post on Twitter."

Ben, like Olivia about 100 pounds overweight, went on to explain: "It's kind of my way to stay connected to Olivia. . . . It's like being there with her." If you're not familiar with the concept of the show, let me explain a little: While taping the show—which is a contest to see who can lose the most weight—contestants are separated from their families and all their normal routines, so as to break all ties with their normal eating cues. Ben had been separated from his wife for weeks by this point, and following my tweets about what we were eating made him feel a little closer.

Some weeks later, at the season finale, Ben was on hand to watch and cheer for his wife, and he was noticeably thinner. He had lost about 100 pounds! We were so impressed that we put him on the show, both to share in his wife's victory and to show off his own achievement. Later, he told us all how he did it, and why it worked.

"I just followed Bob. I watched his tweets. I listened to what he said *he* ate. I figured, how can I go wrong? This is what the *expert* is eating! And that decluttered everything. It made it incredibly clear to me what mattered and what mattered with my diet. It . . . kind of gave me a set of rules."

Bang! *A set of rules.*

Anyone who's ever dieted knows exactly what Ben meant. Today, like never before, we are bombarded from every direction with health advice—about diet, nutrition, weight loss, exercise, organic or nonorganic, free range or corn-fed. Now add in the daily science and medical news, a lot of which sounds either stunningly obvious (not being obese = good) or ridiculously counter to what we *thought* was correct (fruit juice = not so good), and you've got a jumbo case of Clutter Brain.

Clutter Brain is what happens when you hear so much information about a subject that you can't make solid, reasonable decisions—in this case about what you should eat. It's incredibly paralyzing, and just about every dieter knows what often comes with Clutter Brain: anxiety. And you know what that means: exhaustion, depression, and then bingeing. What else—at least in my experience—relieves stress and anxiety better than, say, pie? A whole pie. Right? Which obviously counteracts the benefits of the advice you were trying to follow in the first place.

So, what if we eliminated the clutter? I began to think. What if I could come up with a list of simple, nonnegotiable rules that the average Jane or Joe can follow in daily life—rules you can always fall back on in a pinch, rules you can use not just when you are trying to lose weight, but for when you are trying to *stay* slender.

Skinny Rules!

I'm certainly not the first guy to say this, but in our modern, information-glutted world, rules matter more than ever. Why? Because our external environment no longer seems to have any firm boundaries, any limits, or any positive cues about when to *stop* consuming *anything*. I mean, there is a reason that people get fat—it's easy and cheap to get high-calorie, tasty food. If you look at statistics, more Americans than ever are eating out (and eating enormous portions), eating bad fast food, drinking huge amounts of high-calorie sodas and "energy" waters, and microwaving endless plastic platters of "convenience" food. All of which, while easy, will also make you fat—fast.

But if you want to be right-sized in body, you've got to get rid of the supersize way of life. Whether you want to lose 20 pounds or 200, what the contestants on *The Biggest Loser* have learned—and taught me—holds true: you've got to make a break. You've got to divorce yourself from the past and find a different way of living. And you can never go back.

Once you accept that, and realize there is no finish line, then you've got a better chance of succeeding. Just like Ben, who not only dropped 100 pounds but, so far, has kept it off.

But wow, Bob, you say, *all I want to do is drop 20 pounds!*

No, I don't think so. C'mon. If "all" you want to do is drop 20 pounds, you'd surely have succeeded by now, given the glut of diet books out there, many of which are pretty good.

No. If you are sitting here reading a diet book by one of the trainers on *The Biggest Loser*, I think you . . . kinda . . . want . . . something . . . a little . . . more . . . than . . . "just" dropping some weight.

You want to *keep* the weight off.

You want a way that makes sense in your real-world daily life.

Something convenient *and* healthy.

Something you can always fall back on.

Something permanent, nonnegotiable, and simple.

That's what I want to do with this book. Think of it as a rule book for your life as a healthy-weight person, a person who can enjoy delicious food in the right portions and be satisfied. Someone who can not only resist all the jumbo colas and supersized fries that get waved in front of our noses, but not even feel tempted by them!

Actually, this isn't *only* a rule book. Part I of the book is "The Skinny Rules"—the twenty principles you need to read, understand, and really try to live by. But then I've also created Part II, "The Skinny Way"—a day-by-day menu plan that will get you through the first thirty days of living by the rules. And Part III, "The Skinny Tools," houses the recipes and tips that you'll be called on to look at, cook, and consume! My intention is to take the guesswork out of losing weight for you. After the first thirty days on the program, you will have lost weight and you'll be more confident in eating and living according to my rules. By then you're likely not going to need all of the handholding I provide in this book. You will be on your way to a skinny life!

Don't get me wrong, it won't always be easy. "Easy" does not work. But it will be liberating. Remember what helped Ben: rules and clear instructions freed him from all the brain clutter. These principles let him make rational eating choices without being anxious.

That said, I'll have you know that I *do* have a heart. I get it that these rules are demanding, and that you don't have superhuman willpower (although you have a lot more than you think!). In the first thirty days especially, following all the rules may seem difficult. And depending on how much you have to lose or how you've been eating in the past, it may indeed be so! You are breaking old habits and building new ones, and that's tough. But back to my goodheartedness: I've devised what I like to call a "step-down method" for what most people feel are the handful of most difficult rules. You'll find them marked with a little sign like this: 🌐 These step-downs will help you move away from an old behavior and toward a new, healthy one a little at a time. Keep in mind that this intermediary step is meant to be temporary. Strive to live the rule all the way!

A NEW WAY TO THINK ABOUT DIETING

Feeling motivated to get started? Not quite so fast. Before we begin, we need to clear the deck of some big myths that might hold you in their sway. These myths are based on old dietary rules, even older nutritional science, and still older ways of thinking. In short, they persist—even though they don't work! My guess is that you'll see your own excuses, rationalizations, and assumptions below. But do yourself a favor and hear me out; understanding where you've been wrong or kidding yourself will help you lose weight for good this time.

YOU SAY: "All I have to do is exercise a lot, and the weight will come off."

I SAY: Well, yes—if you've got about five hours to spare every day. That four-mile walk you take every morning? It burns about 350 calories—not even a small bag of fries at McDonald's. That hour of Pilates or yoga? Ditto—not even equal to a large chai latte at Starbucks.

Believe me, it took a lot to convince me of this. I used to believe I could beat anything off of you in the gym. But exercise alone without diet won't do it. (And remember, you don't have all the advantages of my *Biggest Loser* contestants, who have their own trainers for six hours a day and don't have to work around the logistics of everyday life while they are on the show.)

Don't take my word for it. Not long ago a group of Harvard researchers tracked 1,847 overweight men and women, some of whom just exercised, some of whom only dieted. The findings were clear and, for the exercise-deluded, sobering: *"Our results show that isolated aerobic exercise is not an effective weight loss therapy in these patients."*

Got that? I mean, can 1,847 people be wrong?

YOU SAY: "I'm not going to weigh myself more than once a week because it will discourage me and then I will slip."

I SAY: I might once have told you the same thing; the last thing a dieter needs is to be putting him- or herself down all the time for not losing weight fast enough. Or getting depressed when confronted with the enormity of the task.

But that isn't what happens. It turns out that dieters can take the truth just fine, thank you. I recall one contestant telling me why she weighed herself every day: "Bob, I just need to see something real—a hard fact—and that motivates me. It can be depressing, but I've learned that I can take it." She, like Ben, using my tweets, needed something concrete to go on. Is there any science on the subject? Not tons, but when researchers at the Marshfield Clinic in Wisconsin looked at 1,200 dieters, they found that "frequent *self-weighing* seemed to be most beneficial for obese individuals."

It's OK to weigh yourself often. You can take it. Not kidding.

YOU SAY: "It's all calories in, calories out. What else is there to say?"

I SAY: Well, as it turns out: a lot. Sure, you can't suspend the laws of physics, but you can eat foods that do more for your weight loss than other foods. Until recently there wasn't a lot of research to support that claim; the idea that some calories were not as fattening as other calories was ridiculed. But after collecting data about large groups of people over several decades, we're slowly coming around to a new set of understandings.

The most convincing of these comes from Harvard's famed Nurses' Health Study (all women) and Health Professionals Follow-up Study (all men), which have been following 129,000 nurses and health professionals for two decades now. In 2011, the study's researchers decided to try answering one question: are some foods associated with weight loss even if, over time, we've been *increasing* our intake of them?

The answer stunned a lot of traditionalists. Predictably, increases in fruits and veggies were associated with weight loss, while caloric increases in potato chips were associated with weight gain. The shocker came in the less-intuitive items. Increases in nuts, whole grains, and—usefully for us, as you'll see later—yogurt were associated with substantial weight loss.

No one is quite sure why, but we can guess: these foods don't spike your blood sugar and insulin responses the way other foods do, so they don't make you hungry. Also—and you'll hear me go on and on about this later—they are not supersweet or supersalty foods. They don't tweak your psyche to expect those unhealthy extreme flavors you've been eating for so long. Low-fat and even whole-fat milk turn out to be a *lot* better than all those "healthy" fruit juices for which you're shelling out five bucks a pop. I'll tell you why later. In the meantime, you can take heart that your future eating habits won't be as narrow as you might have imagined.

I mean, how wrong could 129,000 nurses *be*?

YOU SAY: "I'll just cut out all carbs or fat—it's that simple."

I SAY: And completely unrealistic. And, let's face it, kind of depressing. In fact, experience tells me that if you are following a diet that tells you to eliminate *an entire crucial nutrient category*—like carbs or fats—then you're in trouble. That's not something you can sustain; you are absolutely going to gain the weight back.

So cutting something out without replacing it—that won't work. I've had trainees tell me over and over, "You know, Bob, I'm Italian American. There's no way I will cut out lasagna completely. It's part of my family and it's a Sunday tradition. It's part of who I am." And I agree. What I am going to show you is how to eat those foods wisely—and I do not always mean itsy-bitsy portions, either!

YOU SAY: "If I don't eat, I'll lose weight: it's that simple."

I SAY: No. One consistent finding over the years is that, for most people, you've got to eat to lose. Part of this is pure metabolism; to strain an old metaphor, you've got to get the engine going for the engine to use all the extra fuel that's hanging around your waist. Also: you're going to slip if you feel too deprived. And you've got to make breakfast *the* priority meal of the day, avoiding the next bad idea, which is . . .

YOU SAY: "I'll just pick up something light on the way to work."

I SAY: Like what? Some yogurt sprinkled with flax seed and acai berries? Uh-uh. *You* know what it's really going be: a bagel and cream cheese, *low-fat cream cheese,* of course, which has worked so well for you so far. So just get this out of your head. While the yogurt/flax seed/berries combo would be great, I'm guessing those ingredients are not in your cupboard at the moment, so in this book I'll give you something new to put in its place: lots of options for a great and satisfying no-hassle breakfast. Remember, one of the key goals of *The Skinny Rules* is to put you back in control of your diet. We'll start with the first and most important meal of the day.

YOU SAY: "It's always bad to lose a lot of weight quickly."

I SAY: The fact is, if you are otherwise healthy, a brief period of rapid weight loss while dieting is reasonably safe. Yes, there can be problems, the most troubling being gall-stones; but these only happen in about 12 percent of extremely obese patients on very low calorie diets for long periods of time. I'm going to assume that doesn't describe you. If it does, go easy. But generally, if you take a multivitamin, hydrate, and make sure you get enough protein and potassium, you'll be fine. And when you look at the scale, you'll get that added psychological boost to keep going.

GET STARTED!

Now that we've dispensed with the ideas and excuses and rationalizations that I believe have held you back in the past, you're ready to go.

Let's treat this as an adventure.

You're going somewhere great!

PART I

THE SKINNY RULES

s I was working on this book, a number of people who read parts over my shoulder said things like, "Wow, Bob. Those are tough. Don't you think people will get discouraged? Can't you make them just a little easier?"

Eventually, I just blurted out, *"I don't want these rules to be liked, I want them to last!"* Furthermore, they aren't that hard! They may be *new*, a.k.a. foreign, but they are not going to deprive you or confound you or leave you confused. I will make sure of that.

Here's the deal: if you want to lose weight and stay thin, you've got to change your life, and that means changing some basic behaviors. I call them defaults—the behaviors that you have instinctively fallen back on when pressured, just as your computer does when it backs itself up. Automatic computer backup = good. Default behaviors = not so good. These defaults have to change.

What does this entail? It entails taking on a new—and, yes, sometimes rigid—set of rules that will, eventually, make perfect sense, but which at first require a leap of faith.

A leap of faith? Sure. You already do this in other areas of your life, be it the obvious (like religion) or the less obvious (say, in suggesting something totally outside the box at work). Or even taking classes for a profession you believe *may* be the way of the future. Taking a leap of faith requires simply having an open mind and a willing spirit.

Take that leap of faith with me. I know these rules are going to change your life for the better. After following the rules for a month—the time most experts agree is needed to form a new habit—I know that you'll be making good food decisions easily (maybe even mindlessly!), you'll have devised your own recipes using mine as your base, and you'll have figured out what menu combinations make you the happiest.

So I have to ask you to proceed by *trusting my process,* even though it may feel foreign at first. Let's get started.

RULE 1

DRINK A LARGE GLASS OF WATER BEFORE EVERY MEAL—NO EXCUSES!

This has got to be the easiest rule there is. Which is a good place to start. But it's also one of the most important rules there is. You simply must stay hydrated. At a minimum I want you to drink a large glass of water before every meal. But I'd prefer that you drink at least five glasses of water a day, the first one within fifteen minutes of waking.

Now, do I really need to harass you about this? I do. Because during the process of losing weight, nothing is so crucial to your success. Water keeps your organs healthy while you're sweating, keeps food moving through the system, and makes you feel full.

Let me put this plainly: drinking water helps you lose weight. You can see this most vividly in very overweight children. Recently, a group of Israeli researchers examined the resting energy expenditure (REE) of twenty-one obese children. REE refers to the rate at which you burn calories when you are sleeping, watching TV, or just simply sitting there and staring into space. The researchers gave the kids a large serving of cold water, then began measuring the REE every 10 minutes. The reaction was more robust than anticipated. Within 24 minutes, REE began increasing. By 57 minutes, REE had increased by 25 percent, and this effect lasted 40 minutes.

Did you get that? Just by drinking water, your body increases its burning of calories. The scientists estimated that, if you just do this, you'll burn off an extra three pounds over the next year.

That doesn't sound like a lot, but I'll take it. Won't you?

The contestants on *The Biggest Loser* are usually chronically dehydrated, and their collective experience shows another reason to drink lots of water. They are usually pretty big consumers of salt before they come on the show. They eat it unknowingly—in the fried and highly processed foods that are their usual mealtime fare and that helped make them so overweight in the first place—and knowingly; too many of them often add salt to whatever they are served. They are usually eating so much salt that they have begun to mess up the delicate mechanisms of chemical balance so vital to our bodies. When the kidneys are swamped with salt and without adequate liquids, you don't get enough potassium. That and other minerals are absolutely key to weight loss.

And as my private fitness clients have shown me, drinking more water helps in other physical ways as well. When they start conscientiously drinking lots of water, their workouts improve. They get less muscle fatigue, they recuperate faster, and they don't feel groggy in the afternoon.

SIMPLE HYDRATION TIPS

- Make it your premeal policy: drink a large glass of water before every meal. No excuses.
- End the day with preparation for a good start to the next: put a large, full glass of water on your bedstand every night and drink it when you wake up, every morning.
- Get a little extra bang for your effort: mix a pitcher of water with a noncaloric vitamin and mineral supplement. I like ElectroMix (one little packet makes a quart), and having the pitcher all mixed and right in front of you will make it that much easier to pour yourself a glass when you open the fridge at every meal; I usually drink mine when I work out.

RULE 2

DON'T DRINK YOUR CALORIES

Caloric beverages steal your health and they steal great food from you. That's right. They steal it because they are so heavily caloric themselves and will fill you up with all the wrong stuff. Think of the kinds of caloric beverages all around you.

SOFT DRINKS: As you heft one of those cans or buckets of sugar water to your mouth, consider that you are *actually eating the equivalent of what should be your entire lunch.*

I came to this rule while working on *TBL*. When I reviewed their pre-*TBL* meal plans I saw that most contestants were drinking Big Gulps or other massive jugs of soda that had 500 calories. Some people would nurse several of them during the day (that's upwards of 1,500 calories of soda a day!). Think of it this way: all that corn syrup? It's a bushel of corn! And remember, when factory farms want to fatten their cattle, what do they do? They feed them corn. So if you are drinking things with corn syrup, think about that. Are you a cow? No you are not.

Moreover, when you drink soda, you are ingesting what just

about every legitimate medical authority in the world has named as suspect number one in today's sprawling diabetes epidemic. A friend of mine tells me that his teenage kids really got the message a few years ago when their father was diagnosed. Now, when a family member asks for a soda, they cheerily reply: "Sure. What kind of diabetes do you want?"

Out of the mouths of babes.

If, like most Americans, you are used to drinking lots of liquid calories, cutting out soda might be a tough adjustment. But it's essential that you kick your soda habit ASAP. If you're a full-calorie soda drinker, you're guzzling empty and unsatisfying calories. If you're a diet/zero-calorie soda drinker, you haven't dodged the problem. Hello?! You're guzzling artificial sweeteners and, as you'll hear again and again in this book, I don't think highly of these at all. They only serve to whet your appetite for more sweet! Stop the madness. Kick the habit.

To help wean yourself from your soda habit, start experimenting with other flavored, noncaloric drinks that you can make yourself. Try seltzer water with lime or lemon juice. Stock up on unsweetened, naturally flavored herb teas. Make a quart or so at a time and keep it in the refrigerator to go with your afternoon snack. And there is my tried-and-true alternative—the "soda eliminator" described in Rule 15. Check it out.

JUICES AND JUICE DRINKS: Most juices have exactly the same number of calories—and the same amount of simple sugars—as a cola. Oh, you'll protest, but doesn't the fiber in a "natural" juice obviate that problem? No. That's just what you've been told. It is the same as drinking a soft drink. You want fruit? Eat fruit.

The whole piece of fruit. Not the extracted and manipulated juice.

Yeah, well, juice smoothies are healthy, right? Maybe "healthy" if you order one with no preservatives or added sugar, but regardless, fruit smoothies that you haven't made yourself (i.e., you have controlled the portions and know exactly what's gone in it) will make you as fat as a Macy's Thanksgiving Day Parade float—just like a 32-ounce soda.

ENERGY REPLACEMENT DRINKS: Well, yeah—if you're training for a marathon. Otherwise, look at the label! A 20-ounce sports drink—let's face it, that's how much you'll "need" to quench that big thirst—weighs in at 130 calories. Like a 12-ounce cola, but without the nifty zing of bubbles and caffeine. I've always seen drinks like these as particularly insidious, because they are, in our heads at least, deeply associated with sports, which are deeply associated with health and fitness. You have to break that connection.

ARTIFICIAL SWEETENERS

Though the scientific jury is still out on whether there is a direct relationship between consuming artificial sweeteners and the urge to eat more sweet-tasting things, I know this from experience with clients, with *The Biggest Loser* contestants, and with myself: the more "sweet" you eat, the more you want it. Another way to put it: when you taste sweet (even the tiny-calorie, artificial kind), you are conditioning yourself to continue wanting and even craving that same sweetness. That continued craving isn't going to help you lose weight—ever. The biggest favor you can do yourself is to leave your sweet consumption to your splurge meal and learn to keep sweet indulgences in perspective: they are treats, not everyday affairs.

A LATTE ON THE WAY TO THE GYM? Sorry. Milk also has a tanker-full of calories. True, coffee itself—which most of the world drinks without milk, by the way—is turning out to be a positive dietary element, although it's still unclear why and how much. I'll get back to that later, but for now, no lattes or chais, frappes, or mochas. If you must get something Euro, get a cappuccino, which contains very little milk (if made the right way), or even an Americano, in which you can better control the amount of milk. And if you must add milk, opt for the low- or no-fat varieties. No cream. No half and half. Whole milk? No again.

ALCOHOL: Although it might sound odd, if there's one source of liquid calories that warrants some leeway in my no-sweetened-beverage world, it's booze. Wine, particularly red wine, deserves a place on your shelf—and on your table. But not when you are trying to *lose* weight! Until you are at your goal weight, it's best to view alcohol the same way you would a Big Gulp. When you get to your goal, red wine is the thing. When you've kept to your goal, we'll talk beer.

> In the same way I want you to step down from soda, I want you to immediately lay off the cream or half-and-half in your coffee. Don't even go for the whole milk. Step down, step away! Start putting 2% milk or nonfat (skim) milk in your coffee and ordering any coffee-based drink that way too. Today.

Now, why am I so down on liquid calories? Most of us know the basics: sugary drinks contain, uh, sugar, and sugar is made up of molecules that encourage the formation of new fat cells, as well as keeping existing ones filled. This applies to *all* sugars, from "natural" ones like honey and juices, to the twin demon spawn of white sugar and high fructose corn syrup. Sugars drive up your blood sugar, which tells the pancreas to make more insulin, which makes you hungry, setting the whole process in motion again.

But what if I told you this: humans are *simply not built* to consume liquid calories.

Period.

That's the growing consensus among nutritionists and medical researchers. In "A Short History of Beverages and How Our Body Treats Them," obesity experts led by the preeminent Barry Popkin scrutinized our evolutionary history and tried to explain why our modern bodies handle them so poorly. Why, for example, do liquid calories make it difficult for our bodies to gauge when they are satisfied, or when to stop eating? After looking at the bodily effects of everything from beer to pop, they put forward a stunning conclusion:

"First," they write, "humans may lack a physiological basis for processing carbohydrate or alcoholic calories in beverages because only breast milk and water were available for the vast majority of our evolutionary history. Alternatives to those two beverages appeared in the human diet no more than 11,000 years ago, but Homo sapiens evolved between 100,000 and 200,000 years ago. Second, carbohydrate and alcohol-containing beverages may produce an incomplete satiation sequence which prevents us from becoming satiated on these beverages."

Translation: when you drink lots of liquid calories, you're fighting 200,000 years of human history!

You're not going to win.

WHY I DRINK COFFEE

Mainly, because I like it! That rich, complex bundle of flavors and smells is comforting and arousing. It makes me happy. But the latest research shows that coffee—in moderation—seems to have all kinds of other benefits as well. Consuming a couple cups (black) a day is strongly tied to lower rates of diabetes, more robust anti-inflammatory gene expression, and better and clearer thinking. It's unclear why coffee does this, but one obvious suspect is caffeine. It is a stimulant, and stimulants generally dampen appetite and increase calorie burning. But . . . I drink it because I like it. As the smell of it wafts into my nostrils, I can close my eyes and envision being in Paris, which is a terrific image. Outside of France, here are some guidelines:

- Drink espresso or black Americano only. Just do it! If you want a cappuccino, opt for nonfat or soy milk in the preparation. That's how I enjoy mine.
- Limit consumption to two cups a day, preferably before noon. Exception: you can drink it all day if you are indeed in Paris.
- Decaf espresso is fine after lunch until around five. After that even the small amounts of caffeine will disturb your sleep.

RULE 3

EAT PROTEIN AT EVERY MEAL—OR STAY HUNGRY AND GROUCHY

n my world, protein—in almost all forms—reigns; for dieters it is the key food group. Simply put, you've got to eat more—at least a lot more than the FDA (Food and Drug Administration) currently tells you.

But why at every meal? Because:

1. You will get the satisfaction and hunger-reducing benefits sprinkled throughout your day. (You don't want to get hungry at two o'clock, and you can prevent that by eating protein at lunch.)
2. If you weigh 200 pounds, I want you to get at least 100 grams of protein a day (see the box for some *TBL* faves); you're not going to do that in one meal. Spread it out over three meals and you'll have no trouble. And . . .
3. Almost all forms of protein taste great; eating it at every meal gives you a chance to make your menu more diverse and less boring, which is pretty important to a dieter.

But remember, not all calories are equal, and so it is with protein. To my mind, fish is the Protein King. You can't get a better, more satisfying dish. Let me be blunt: if you don't start eating fish, you're going to get fat again. Given that, let's start there with our discussion of how to add protein to your repertoire.

FISH

But Bob, you'll say, we don't eat fish in our household. Well, we didn't in ours, either—but that may have been because I grew up in Tennessee and we didn't have a grasp of the fundamentals of healthy fish preparation. (It's not complicated—I'll get to that in "The Skinny Tools"). I suspect the same is true for a lot of people. But don't let having been raised in a house where fish was not part of the weekly lineup be an excuse to carry on that insane tradition!

After you find out about all of its benefits, I'm hopeful you'll be a convert.

Let's start with the benefit you are most interested in: weight loss. Like we talked about in the beginning, some foods seem to boost weight loss—and not just because they are low in calories. Fish is a perfect example. If you look at groups of people on identical diets—except for how much fish they eat—you see something remarkable. The dieters eating fish lose about a kilogram (about 2.2 pounds) more than their fellows over the same period of time. That is what a group of Icelandic researchers found when they subjected four groups of men (totaling 324 participants) to four different diets of the same caloric and nutrient levels. The ones who got the most fatty fish lost the most weight. That led the researchers to conclude that "the addition of seafood to a nutritionally balanced energy-restricted diet may boost weight loss."

The key to so much of the attention fish gets these days has to do with something you've likely heard a lot about: omega-3 fatty acids and their benefits in preventing or treating chronic disease. Let me do a short—and, I hope, painless—primer for you, so you'll know why I will keep harping on this.

Omega-3s are what nutritionists call essential fatty acids. Fatty acids are made up of a chain of carbon (and sometimes hydrogen) atoms, and they are a backbone of your body's ability to make fuel for itself. They convert raw, unusable fuel into a refined, high-octane energy source. But—the body doesn't make essential fatty acids. It has to get them via what you eat. And fish has them in spades.

It turns out that omega-3s have all kinds of other benefits. It's unclear what the exact mechanisms are, but a lot of it boils down to how omega-3s control inflammation, which you might as well get a grip on now too, because this topic is *the* player in today's attempts to control chronic disease.

Briefly, inflammation is your body's defense system; when something foreign invades—bacteria, some bad air—your liver and pancreas begin to generate all kinds of warrior chemicals that kill the bad guy. That's why you don't get a huge infection and gangrene when you get a cut; you get some redness, some heat, some pain, some swelling—all signs that your inflammatory system is doing its job. The problem is when this powerful system is sent into overdrive too often—by bad foods, among other things. That's why we get plaques on our arteries, and that's why those plaques sometimes "blow up" and cause a heart attack or stroke. It's also one reason that blood sugar gets out of control, which leads to diabetes, blindness, nerve damage, and limb amputation.

Fortunately, our bodies have a natural check on this disastrous chain—*if* we get enough omega-3 fatty acids. They act as a kind of selective fire extinguisher—they tamp down inflammatory particles when we don't need them. We can get a lot of omega-3s from capsules, liquids, and tablets—which is great, although trickier if you are using certain prescription drugs that might minimize their effect. Then there is the safer and tastier option: fish, particularly salmon and albacore tuna. (If just reading those two words makes you think "boring," get ready to change your mind—I've got some easy recipes for you later.) The list of benefits is growing every day—from improved cholesterol, blood pressure, and blood sugar to bone health and muscle protection.

All of that is great—but how does fish help me lose weight, you ask?

I like to say that I always feel lighter when I have eaten fish—and I don't mean as in "empty stomach." In fact, I feel full longer but not heavy or sluggish. The young science of satiety—the study of food satisfaction—tells us that some combination of proteins and fats in fish is responsible for this benefit. The other reason is pure volume: just look at how big one 6-ounce serving of tilapia looks compared to the same amount of steak. It's huge. If you use some of the recipes in Part III I guarantee you will be full and happy—but not fat.

JUST HOW MUCH PROTEIN IS ENOUGH PROTEIN?

The official answer is: no one really knows. The FDA says protein should be 10 percent of your total daily calories. The National Research Council says 8 percent. The National Academy of Sciences: 6 percent. I'm going to give you what we might call the Skinny Recommendation: take your weight and divide it by two—that's how much protein you should be eating in grams every day. If you're 200 pounds, try to get at least 100 grams. I'm not saying it's 100 percent scientific, but more and more research shows that consumption of a high-protein diet with reduced high-carb foods results in better weight control metabolism. I'm saying it works. For me. For my clients, my contestants, and for you.

ANIMAL PROTEIN AND ME

Some of you who've read about me in the last several years and thought I was vegan will be surprised to see that I recommend animal proteins at all. There's a personal story behind this.

The "compassion" argument was a big part of my decision to go vegan—I care about the treatment of animals, and I've read and seen the films about the conditions at many farms and slaughterhouses. I have also read about the health and disease-prevention benefits of reducing or swearing off animal proteins. *The China Study* by T. Colin Campbell is one of the most convincing studies there could be. Campbell studied Asian eating patterns for decades, and the results of his work showed in great detail that some of today's healthiest populations are those that do not eat meat.

So, I went vegetarian, then vegan. No animal protein for me! Milk—no, I'll take a soy latte or a soy cheese. An omelet? Only if you make it with scrambled tofu. There were veggie burgers and almond loafs and enough dal and lentils and curries and falafels to fill a stadium. It worked: my cholesterol went down. I lost weight. I felt lighter. For me, being strictly vegan was work—I scrutinized everything I ate—but my health was clearly worth the effort.

But after a few years, the benefits start to wane. I was fatigued. And I was getting . . . soft, which is not a particularly good thing if you are the trainer for a show called *The Biggest Loser.* My own trainer, Sam Upton (who has, let's say, the perfectly fit body—the kind that trainers themselves strive for!), suggested I needed to reintroduce some animal protein to regain my muscle tone and strength.

My own experience isn't scientific but it is significant—bringing some animal protein back into my diet helped my energy levels. I stayed lean. I felt better.

I am a reluctant omnivore, I have to admit. I still have all the reservations about meat, about the way the animals are treated, and about its health effects. But I also believe that we are quickly changing the way we treat animals—free range has become a mainstream concept; we pass laws to make sure our animals have better living quarters; and slowly but surely, even the meat industry is getting the message about better animal husbandry and hygiene. Slowly, yes. But it's happening. And we can take advantage of those changes for our own benefit. And for the animals: if we demand cruelty-free food, we'll create a market for it, and thus encourage farmers to continue such improvements. The power of the eater's purse is remarkable. Use it, I say.

I still very much advocate a plant-based diet for the most part. You'll see in my menus and recipes, I don't ever recommend that anyone go heavy on the animal protein, but I also don't think it is so awful to eat a steak or a breast of chicken or some cheese in an otherwise plant-heavy regimen. The country's most lauded vegan chef, Tal Ronnen, was recently interviewed on just this conundrum. His response? "So be a vegan who eats bacon!"

EGGS . . .

. . . to the rescue! Here's a fun fact for you: I eat a half dozen egg whites a day. That's because they are 20 calories apiece, a saving of 60 calories an egg without the yolks and an amazing source of protein. But whether you use just the white or the whole thing, eggs are versatile. They can make a boring soup tasty, or a dinner salad so satisfying you'll want to go out and get your own chickens! They are a kind of magic food, in that they seem to make everything else taste richer.

I have also discovered that, if you put just one yolk into a five-egg-white omelet, you get a nice yellow color and a deeper taste. I make it for my contestants and they love it—even the egg white haters! Note: get the omega-3 eggs if you can.

CHICKEN AND TURKEY

The modern dieter's default food, poultry (especially chicken breast), is a useful tool in your weight-loss cabinet, and we'll use it, but don't think every day. I do not want you to get bored—boredom leads to loss of focus on your goal: weight loss!

A few poultry notes: again, I prefer organic. Maybe even more important are things like "humanely raised," "free range," and "sustainably farmed." This I recommend not just for eco-reasons, but because you are going to get a tastier bird, and when you're three weeks into a weight-loss program, taste matters.

But when in doubt, remember fish—it's better than both beef and poultry!

PORK

The "other white meat" is not one of my favorites. I think pork producers have a long way to go in improving their treatment of the animals, and furthermore, the pork products we find at the supermarket are too often dry, tasteless, and tough. That said, I also know you need diversity in your diet. Fortunately, slowly but surely, we're finding more pork producers who take pride in their humane treatment of animals. The best of these is the famed Niman Ranch, the California producers who've become the go-to favorite of big-time chefs around the country (and Niman Ranch products are now available in many local supermarkets too). Pork from such producers tends to be juicier and tastier. Which cuts? Loin is lowest in calories, the rump the highest in fat. Use the former as a replacement for chicken.

BEEF

Remember, because of density and mass, a serving of fish is likely going to look and feel a whole lot more satisfying than 6 ounces of beef. But assuming you want to have some variety and/ or can't get your head around a diet without beef, you simply need to keep some things in mind so you don't lose perspective.

As with almost all animal protein, I prefer that you go organic and grass fed. It's more expensive, I know, I know. But since you are going to be eating beef more selectively and strategically, you may find you can afford it—or at least *some* of it—in organic form. Organic is not a blanket commandment with me. If you don't have any organic meat in your refrigerator and it's dinnertime, eat the nonorganic meat. This is about reasonable, healthy weight loss first.

That said, there are many benefits to, say, grass fed. It's got a ton of those wonderful omega-3 fatty acids, and a lot of—sorry to get technical—conjugated linoleic acid, or CLA. Like omega-3, CLA is a molecule produced by the body as part of the normal metabolic cycle, but as it turns out, it also aids in weight control. There have been thirty-five studies on this aspect of CLA so far. The general wisdom: CLA—which is found only in beef (OK, and *kangaroo meat*)—helps reduce body fat and increase lean mass. I'll take that!

Stick with the leanest cuts (see the box on beef cuts). I want you to cook them simply, with no sauces (except at your splurge meal). And I want you to pay attention to appropriate serving sizes! Rule 9 will tell you what you need to know and, again, I think you'll find it interesting to see that a serving size of lean steak is a *lot* smaller than other forms of protein. So, it's your call—more of other kinds of proteins or less steak. Of course, more food will make you feel more satisfied. I mean, when you have to decide between one itsy beef burger or two turkey burgers, I think I know which one you'll pick. Besides, turkey is probably a better go-to protein than beef if you're serious about weight loss. And you are. You are seriously serious.

CUTS OF BEEF

Leanest

CUT (lean, trimmed)	CALORIES per 4 ounces (cooked)
Eye of round steak	188
Sirloin tip side steak	197
Bottom round steak	225
Top round steak	226
Top sirloin steak	247

Fattiest

CUT (lean, trimmed)	CALORIES per 4 ounces (cooked)
New York strip steak	232
Filet mignon	261
Skirt steak	286
Porterhouse steak	320
T-bone steak	320
Rib-eye steak	322

CHEESE

Cheese—the right one at the right time (and in moderation)—
has its benefits. Many varieties are low in calories, high in protein,
and devoid of carbohydrates. Just as important for anyone who
wants to achieve *lasting* weight loss, cheese is versatile. You can
make breakfasts, snacks, desserts, and even dinner with it. You can
use cheese (such as parmesan) as a condiment to flavor a dish,
as a topping (think ricotta or feta) to complete partial proteins
(like beans), or just because it tastes and looks so good! My favorites are goat cheese, mild cheddar, feta, blue, and parmesan
cheese.

You might note that I have no objections to some full-fat
cheeses. What can I say? A great cheddar is a great cheddar, and
even an ounce is amazingly satisfying. I have a favorite snack: a
little hummus, a few Persian cucumbers (the smaller, thinner-
skinned variety now found in most stores), and a small piece of
hard cheese. I take pictures of it, I love it so much!

TOFU AND TEMPEH

Last but not least, there are the nonanimal proteins of tofu and
tempeh. There was a time when products like these were considered "alternative" proteins—replacements for cheese or meat for
vegans and vegetarians. But today, like vegetarianism and even
veganism, tofu and tempeh have gone mainstream. These ingredients are easy to find in almost every grocery store, they show up on
restaurant menus all over the country, and they are fast becoming
part of the cooking repertoire for non-vegans/non-vegetarians too
(especially tofu). And they are not hard to cook—see my recipes
for some tasty options.

A 3.5-ounce serving of tofu, made of coagulated soy milk, has 75 calories and 8.1 grams of protein. Tempeh, a denser (thus its smaller serving size), fermented version of tofu, weighs in at 160 calories and 15 grams per half-cup serving. Use them on your meatless day!

RULE 4

SLASH YOUR INTAKE OF REFINED FLOURS AND GRAINS

Grains—mainly in the form of refined flours—dominate our modern diet. Pasta is king. Bagels are everyday. Grains in all kinds of shapes and sizes are cheap and tasty and everywhere.

They might be marketed as "low in fat," "all natural," "whole," and even "heart healthy." But if they are at all refined—from rice to bread—they make you fat.

That's because grains are a lot like liquid calories once your body processes them. Remember Dr. Popkin's observation in Rule 2? As with liquid calories, throughout our evolutionary history, we didn't eat them. We were not built to eat them, or at least a lot of them. Only relatively recently have grains become a substantial, routine part of our diet. And like liquid calories, our endless consumption of them comes with a huge health care bill, from diabetes to irritable bowel syndrome to heart disease, as well as skin rashes, immune-system disorders, and, of course, the new specter, gluten allergies.

Does this mean you will never again savor spaghetti with clam sauce? Are we done with burritos? Maybe more important, you ask: how can I live without something in my diet that is as comforting and satisfying as white rice, white bread, or even cornmeal?

This concern might have served as a legitimate barrier only a few years back, but the supermarket and specialty store shelves increasingly offer tasty alternatives that I have come to love. And they don't make me soft.

Before we get to that, let me take you on a brief and, I think, surprising tour of the science of refined and whole grains.

Refined grains—as the first one on the label is often "wheat flour" on the label—started out almost literally as a breakfast of kings. When all the peasants were gnawing their way through amaranth and boiled wheat berries, the rich could afford to get someone to strip off all that bran and make a beautifully soft-textured bread, which became all the rage. As modern food technology made this process affordable to Jane and Joe Average, it also took away the two most important parts of the kernel—the bran and the germ. The former is utterly indispensable for digestion, and the latter brings nutrients by the bushel. What is left is, literally and metaphorically, an empty husk.

But it is a dangerous empty husk. Without the bran, starchy carbs get stuck in our gut for much longer than they should, and begin to interrupt normal bodily processes. Healthy bacteria get starved. Starchy carbs without much nutritive value depress important hormones that cause you to feel full, and they stimulate hormones that make you hungry. And without the germ, you get nothing in terms of minerals and vitamins and protein. By the time these carbs get processed in your liver, you have a time bomb of sugar that sends blood sugar and insulin up, and that much-desired feeling of fullness . . . down, down, down.

By contrast, whole grains have huge benefits: they speed up digestion, increase good hormones and decrease bad hormones, steady blood sugar and insulin, drive up satiety, and, in short, make weight gain just a little less likely. The work of Dr. Inger Björck, of Sweden's Lund University, is a case in point. Björck, who comes from a long line of diabetics, was fascinated with one idea: does the gut have a memory? In other words, are there ways to stimulate our gut lining to "remember" to healthfully process food? Björck tried an experiment. Some patients she had eat a very small serving of barley with their evening meal; other patients ate the same meal without the barley. In the morning, researchers drew blood samples and measured blood sugar levels. The barley eaters' were better.

That was hardly shocking. "What was surprising is what happened next," says Björck. "We fed both groups a nice hearty breakfast, with eggs, toast, and even bacon. Two hours later we measured blood sugar again. What we found is that the barley eaters still had a low blood sugar reading! It was as if the gut had been reprogrammed." The effect lasted until well after lunch. Barley eaters reported feeling full. "There maybe is such a thing as gastric memory," she says. "And our job is to find ways to stimulate it to remember the right ways to process our foods."

Yes, yes, yes, you say. But do you think that I, with three kids, a job, and a dog to walk really have time to soak and rinse and boil grains to make them edible? No, you don't have that kind of time. But you do have twenty minutes on a Sunday evening, don't you? That's all it really takes for many whole grains, from farro—an ancient Italian strain of wheat that fed Hannibal when he crossed the Alps (FYI: Hannibal was not fat)—to barley, which does not need to be soaked.

If you are really going to abide by this rule—and I believe it is utterly essential to your success at losing weight and keeping it off—you've got to learn to read labels. (See Rule 8 for more on that activity!) Especially on bread. Here is the most important tip: if the nutritional information on a loaf of bread does not *lead* with the words "*whole-grain* wheat flour" or "sprouted whole wheat," pass it by. I don't care if the colorful "down-home" label says it is "multigrain," "nutty," "whole wheat," "natural," "stone ground," or whatever! If it doesn't say, first and foremost, "whole-grain wheat flour," then just keep on walkin'. Ditto if *any* sweetener appears within the first five ingredients. If you take just a little more time in your regular supermarket to read labels, you'll soon know which breads and grains are rule-abiding.

What if you *don't* have twenty minutes, or you are just feeling lazy? Fortunately, there are still some great options. Whole-grain pastas that *are actually tasty* can now be found in lots of mainstream grocery stores. They are an amazing source of fiber—*9 grams per serving at only 200 calories*. But when shopping for and preparing pasta, pay attention. Take note:

1. There should be two things in the ingredients: whole-wheat flour (or whole-wheat durum flour) and water. That's it. Whole-wheat pasta has 9 grams of fiber versus 2 in regular!

2. A serving size is one-eighth of a pound, or 2 ounces. If you're preparing spaghetti or other long, thin pastas (linguini, angel hair, etc.), here's a rule of thumb: make an "OK" sign as big as a dime—that's a serving size. What about shapes like penne and fusilli? Again, an eighth of a pound. Imagine an eighth of the one-pound bag or box. Or, for the first two or three times, weigh out the portion for future reference. And that's it— 200 calories. OK? Pasta is meant to rest underneath another kind of food—veggies, I say (see #6 below)! It's not meant to be the main ingredient!

3. When you cook the pasta, do it in a big pot, and test it several

times for doneness. It should be just a tad al dente, which means slightly hard or underdone in the center.

4. When you drain the pasta, don't rinse it. That's so un-Italian! The natural glutens left on the pasta will make your sauce stick to the noodles.

5. Save about ¼ cup of the pasta water to add to the sauce at the last minute—an old country trick that kicks up the taste and enriches the sauce without adding calories.

6. Try eating your serving of pasta with as many sautéed or braised greens as you like. Use olive oil—no more than a tablespoon—to cook down the greens. Toss the greens and the pasta together; don't just pile them on top. Now you're at 350 calories—one fifth of your daily allotment. With 4 ounces of salmon: 550!

7. Use that parmesan cheese. Great taste, and it takes the place of salt.

8. Eat pasta at lunch (see Rule 7) instead of dinner when you can.

Looking for other grains? Allow me to introduce you to farro! For decades health food folk have been soaking whole wheat berries to make them edible. Only the most committed persist for any substantial length of time; the benefit/effort ratio doesn't pan out. But what if you could get the benefits of whole wheat berries without the hassle and *with* some extra taste? That's why I recommend farro, a version of wheat that has been used by Italians since the Roman Empire. Farro gives you a whopping 7 grams of protein and 3 grams of fiber (brown rice nets only 2) per serving. It takes just twenty minutes to make if you use the semipearled variety and you can get it at many supermarkets, at your local Italian deli, or online. It tastes nutty and rich. It will change the way you think about whole wheat forever. See pages 226 and 227 for recipes.

In the bread category, there is one great brand out there that I eat and recommend all the time: Ezekiel bread. Made with no flour (it is made from grains and sprouts), Ezekiel bread comes in many varieties—from cinnamon raisin to sesame to wheat—and you'll usually find it in the freezer section of your store. It has a bit more "chew" than bread you might be used to, but that extra heartiness will likely mean you'll not eat as much of it as you might of other, lighter, less healthy breads.

"Wow, Harper," you might be thinking. "No white bread and no white grains? OK. But what about brown rice? I don't see you talking about that a lot."

It's true that nutritionists, diet gurus, and macramé vendors have long advocated this "miracle grain" as a replacement for white rice. But hardheaded nutritional science suggests otherwise. A portion of brown rice offers only one more gram of fiber than does white rice (2 grams versus 1). Its protein advantage is also negligible. And while it is true that brown rice has a lot more micronutrients and vitamins than white rice, those increased amounts are negligible when it comes to meeting your daily requirements.

But I told you I have a heart. I'm not going to take this away from you quite yet. Try using brown rice when you must, no more than ½ cup at a time; it's a step down from white rice to be sure. Make the swap immediately but aim to wean yourself from rice entirely—there are so many great grains from which to choose a replacement.

If I were you I'd cook up four servings on Sunday evening, let them cool, and put in individual bags for later in the week. You can also find premeasured and precooked packets in the market now. These you can simply pop into the microwave and eat. But never more than ½ cup!

RULE 5

EAT 30 TO 50 GRAMS OF FIBER A DAY

Our highly processed "convenient" food supply doesn't supply any fiber. Or very little. So you've got to make a special commitment to finding foods that have it, and to eating it regularly. That's why most of the other must-eat recommendations in *The Skinny Rules* have a lot of fiber. You're going to get those 30 to 50 grams if I have to come over there and put them in your yogurt myself!

Let's get schooled. There are two different kinds of fiber. The first, soluble fiber, is just that. It gets dissolved by water and absorbed into the bloodstream, where cells use its various components for vital functions. It comes mainly from plants—fruits, vegetables, beans, nuts, oat bran, barley, flax.

The second is *in*soluble fiber. This kind doesn't break down like the other; it can't get into cells so remains in the digestive system, where it keeps food moving, sweeps clean the gastrointestinal tract, and signals a bunch of antihunger molecules. It comes from wheat bran, rice bran, and corn bran, and from the skins of fruits and veggies, nuts, seeds, and whole-grain foods.

For decades, you've been hearing all kinds of health claims about fiber: it lessens the risk of colorectal cancer, drives down bad cholesterol, and prevents the onset of type 2 diabetes, the scourge of modern life. There are varying levels of data about the first two claims—generally positive—but the findings about diabetes, weight loss, and fiber are increasingly compelling and worthy of just a moment of your time.

Type 2 diabetes—called "adult onset" diabetes until obese high school students started presenting with it—is the condition your Southern grandmother might have called "the sugar," or "my sugar." (*"Oh, I can't eat the pecan pie—it's bad for my sugar, baby!"*) It's anything but grandmotherly to your body. When you repeatedly tax your muscles to take in more sugar, they eventually become resistant to the gatekeeper hormone insulin, made by the pancreas. So the insulin and excess sugar go packing off into the bloodstream, where they inflame skin, muscle, heart, and nerve cells. Foot infections, accelerated skin aging, and eye disease are common. You get dark circles under your eyes and elbows that turn scaly black. In patients with uncontrolled diabetes, blindness and amputation are not uncommon outcomes. I mean, it says something when—in small and large cities—*preventing amputation* is a key public health priority.

Eating fiber in the amounts I'm advocating is looking more and more promising as a way to prevent type 2. And I am talking fiber from *food*, not from supplements. An extensive review by researchers at the Technical University of Dresden, for example, noted that the development of type 2 diabetes mellitus can even be prevented by dietary changes. They wrote: "A low-fat diet with a dietary fiber intake of more than 30g/d was shown to represent an effective preventive approach."

What are the benefits of fiber intake for weight loss? We already know the basic mechanisms of the process—gastrointestinal "sweeping," satiety signals, increased feelings of being full, and so on—but what can we expect, weight-loss wise, from boosting our fiber intake? One of the best ways to get a handle on that is to look once again at studies of whole grain. To date, there have been fourteen large, cross-sectional studies of whole-grain consumption in the United States. As reported in a recent nutrition journal, "A higher intake of whole grains (a daily intake of ~3 servings) is associated with lower BMI [body mass index] in adults." Three studies found that adults who upped how much whole grain they ate had smaller waist circumferences. And the Baltimore Longitudinal Study of Aging reported *an inverse association* between whole-grain consumption and body mass index, as well as, perhaps more important, waist-to-hip ratio and waist circumference. The most likely weight-loss component of the grain is, you guessed it, fiber.

In my Tweets and Facebook posts, I often go on and on about my fiber rule. Why? Because I have witnessed so many bodily transformations that would never have been possible without it. I can't emphasize it enough.

If you follow my rules *you just can't help but get enough fiber without getting too many calories.* And in case you don't have time to sit down for a meal, I have a meal replacement drink that will get you 14 grams by itself (see page 188). Because it is so full of nutrients—and so low in calories and sugars—it's one of the few drinkable-calorie menu items I can recommend.

MY TOP DELICIOUS SOURCES OF FIBER

Fruits (skin on!)

Apples:	1 medium	=	4 grams
Blueberries:	½ cup	=	2 grams
Peaches:	1 medium	=	2.3 grams
Pears:	1 medium	=	5.5 grams
Raspberries:	½ cup	=	3.5 grams
Strawberries:	½ cup sliced	=	9 grams

Vegetables

Acorn squash:	½ cup cubed	=	4.5 grams
Broccoli:	½ cup	=	2 grams
Brussels sprouts:	1 cup	=	4 grams
Cabbage:	1 cup	=	5.5 grams
Carrots:	½ cup	=	3.4 grams
Cauliflower:	1 cup	=	3 grams
Spinach:	1 cup	=	7 grams
Zucchini:	1 cup	=	8 grams

Breads, Cereals, and Beans

Black-eyed peas:	¼ cup	=	4.5 grams
Ezekiel bread:	1 slice	=	3.5 grams
Garbanzo beans:	¼ cup	=	3.5 grams
Kidney beans:	¼ cup	=	4 grams
Lima beans:	¼ cup	=	3.5 grams
Plain oatmeal:	½ cup	=	2 grams
Whole-grain pasta:	2 ounces dry	=	6.3 grams

RULE 6

EAT APPLES AND BERRIES
EVERY SINGLE DAY. EVERY.
SINGLE. DAY!

This rule sounds so airy, fluffy, easy. Right? But it's just as important as the rest, and if you want to make weight loss permanent, you'd better avail yourself of these delicious fruits. I do.

When visitors come over to my house, they are likely to find me at work at my dining-room table, snacking on fruits: apples (sometimes by themselves, sometimes with a small piece of cheese or some peanut butter); strawberries and blueberries (maybe with some Greek yogurt; see my Skinny Shake recipe on page 187); or raspberries and blackberries (alone, or on my oatmeal in the morning).

I love these snacks. To me they taste like fruit *should* taste: sweet but not too much so, and bursting with complex flavor, a little tangy, a little herbal, a little tingly on the tongue, and, most important, satisfying.

That sounds like I am describing my beloved evening red wine! And in many ways it should.

Because in recent years their scientific storylines have run in parallel. As in the case of wine, some of the world's leading nutrition experts have discovered all kinds of benefits in these and other common and tasty fruits. Some of their findings are obvious to almost anyone who follows the nation's endless drool of health "news": they have lots of desirable vitamins (C and E), all kinds of micronutrients (folic acid, selenium, beta carotene), and lots of fiber, which by now you know I consider absolutely key to sustained weight loss.

But other findings are revealing a whole new side to these everyday (or *should* be everyday) fruits. It's worth just a few minutes of your time to understand what's going on. . . .

Apples and berries are rich in a class of natural molecules called phytochemicals. In the human body, these are usually involved in some stage of metabolism. Some of them inhibit certain processes, others speed it. The most important phytochemicals, for our purposes, are anthocyanins, usually concentrated in the skin of colorful fruits and vegetables.

Anthocyanins, along with other phytochemicals like quercitin and ellagitannins, seem to act as powerful natural anti-inflammatories. Better, they seem to push down bad cholesterol and its harmful effect on the heart and arteries. In fact, when you track groups of people consuming *in*creased amounts of berries over time, you can see an actual *de*crease in deaths from heart attacks. And if you take a blood sample from someone who has ingested apples and berries, you see better blood sugar control: another example of gastric memory.

I'd like to note here, for anyone concerned about the aesthetic effects of aging, that these molecules are also under intense study for their favorable effect on the skin. And, of course, you don't have to buy them from some expensive store selling anti-aging cosmetics and supplements hawked by some Beverly Hills doctor. The best way to get phytochemicals is to eat them!

But what about these fruits *and weight loss*? Outside of the obvious—they are low in calories and high in fiber—is there something unique about them that makes them better for losing weight than other foods?

The nutrition scholar Barbara Rolls—perhaps the preeminent expert on how humans process bulky and fibrous foods—had exactly this question in mind when, a few years ago, she came up with an experiment. For five weeks, she gave fifty-eight patients one of three meal "preloads," each containing 125 calories. One group got whole apples, one got applesauce, and one got apple juice with "fiber added." (A control group got no preload.) Fifteen minutes after, the subjects were allowed to eat as much as they wanted.

The results were surprising: the subjects who ate the whole apple consistently ate 15 percent less than the subjects in all the other groups. They also stayed fuller longer. All of this led Rolls to conclude something I have been haranguing people about for some time. But let her tell it in her spare, clinical prose: "Overall, whole apple increased satiety more than applesauce or apple juice. Adding naturally occurring levels of fiber to juice did not enhance satiety. These results suggest that *solid fruit affects satiety more than pureed fruit or juice, and that eating fruit at the start of a meal can reduce energy intake*" (emphasis mine).

That's what I said!

The other surprising mechanism through which phytochemicals may make it easier to lose weight concerns germs. More precisely, bacteria in our guts—those friendly bacteria you hear so much about in advertisements for yogurts and probiotic drinks. These are called, as a group, intestinal microbials, and when they are in balance, they help stabilize energy expenditure versus energy storage—what you want to prevent weight gain. However, when you get fat, you throw this balance out of whack—essentially in favor of fat storage. Phytochemicals like those in apples and berries seem to restore the balance. Maybe just as important: the fruits do this job better—and with far fewer calories—than yogurt, soy yogurt, and all those pricey probiotic drinks. In fact, the researchers suggested that one future bacteria supplement for weight loss would use *mainly* fruit phytochemicals and just a *little* bit of yogurt.

I'm not going to wait for the results.

Given all this great nutritional news, it should be easy to go out and find a person who's eating at least two or three fruits a day, like the FDA and other health authorities suggest, right? No. Not in the land of supersweet, superfast, supereverything all the time. Only about one third of adults and *13 percent* of children eat two portions a day. The contestants on *TBL* who do so are the ones who get the weight off and *keep* it off.

But why the reluctance to eat more fruit? Flavor, inconvenience, and price come to mind. Supermarket apples are often crisp, pretty—and flavorless. Berries can be mushy, pulpy, and pricey, the latter of which I am endlessly reminded by my cheapskate writing partner. But you (and he!) might be surprised by a few things. One, frozen berries of all kinds are just as good as fresh berries—as long as there are no added sugars (including juice), and they tend to cost less. They are also convenient, and you can use them in all kinds of treats, from smoothies to fruit salads. What about apples? In the big cities, more and more supermarkets are bringing back all kinds of heirloom varieties long ago abandoned by the industry. They taste great—they actually taste like something other than sugar—and, more and more, they are available organic and locally grown. The latter cost more but, as we'll discuss later, you can choose to be selectively organic in your menu planning.

ORGANIC MUST-BUYS VS. OPTIONAL ORGANICS

"A well-balanced diet can equally improve health regardless of its organic or conventional origin." That's pretty much the scientific consensus about organic food. I mention this because (a) I know I am going to hear about this from a lot of you, (b) I am concerned about cost and availability, and (c) I don't like my trainees to do things out of needless fear. I want you to use your head to make rational decisions to remake your body.

This does not mean that, for various reasons, some foods aren't better organic than others. If you want to pay to play it extra safe, here are some foods worth the extra buck:

Worth-it organics

apples	peaches
asparagus	pears
celery	spinach
cherries	strawberries
lettuce	sweet bell peppers
nectarines	tomatoes

Not-worth-it organics

avocados	kiwifruit
bananas	mangos
broccoli	onions
cabbage	papayas
frozen peas	pineapple

RULE 7

NO CARBS AFTER LUNCH

All my rules are important, but this is a big one because the barrier to pulling it off is as much psychological as it is physical. Why? Because as we work, put up with idiotic bosses and coworkers, sit out traffic jams and suffer through insane public transportation, we begin to feel like we are owed something at the end of the day. Or that we deserve something. And for too many of us, that something is usually based on sugar, whether in the form of simple sugars or starchy carbohydrates.

I don't blame anyone who feels this way.

It's utterly human.

But we have to break that habit, eat most of our carbohydrates in the morning, and live by a different array of foods—proteins and fiber in the afternoon. Let me say this again: aim for lots of protein and fiber after lunch. No or very low carbs, and those only if offset by even more fiber.

You'll see in "The Skinny Tools" that most of my dinner recommendations are high in protein and fiber, so take a look at those options to expand your repertoire of evening meals. I'll also give you some great no-carb snacks later on. But first, focus on the *why*: what happens when you eat carbs late in the day?

Carbs are forms of sugar, and sugar cues the pancreas to make more insulin, which in turn triggers appetite. The later in the day that you consume sugar, the more likely it is that you will get food cravings late at night. Late-night cravings are not a good thing!

The latest research about sugar metabolism has taken this basic insight and built on it. One of the hot buzz-phrases in that research world is "insulin excursions." (It has nothing to do with travel.) It turns out that the *number of times during the day* that you signal your pancreas to make insulin is just as important as how much sugar you eat. Each "excursion" is like a hammer delivering blow after blow to your cells. No wonder today's diabetes experts want you to limit the number of times you eat carbs, especially in the evening. Add to this the fact that insulin cues hunger hormones in the gut, and you've got one incredibly powerful physiological response.

Believe me, you're not going to win that battle if you fight it the conventional way.

But you can strategically manage that war to your own weight-loss benefit. I'll give you two guiding principles:

- Snack on fiber, protein, vegetables, and fresh fruits (not dried fruits).
- Eat lean and green at night.

Repeat. Post on refrigerator door.
If you can abide by this rule, you're gonna be thin.

RULE 8

LEARN TO READ FOOD LABELS
SO YOU KNOW WHAT YOU ARE EATING

I f you are like me you might react to this rule the same way you did a nagging aunt or freshman-year health teacher.

But stop rolling your eyeballs and listen: you've got to do this, because it is going to put you back in control of your food, your diet, your body, and your life. It did this for me and for dozens of my clients and *Biggest Loser* contestants, and it's going to do it for you. Trust my process.

Let's start with the fact that, if you are like most of our fellow Americans (in fact, most earthlings), you are ruled by dietary *mis*-information. Or confusion. Or just plain ignorance. You're not alone. When asked to read the labels of common food items, the majority of consumers often can't figure out the basics. And no wonder. The modern nutrition label is frequently confusing—graphically busy, laden with irrelevant claims and detail, sometimes almost impossible to find on the container. And that's on top of one of my great pet peeves: ridiculously small portion sizes. The heck with that.

Before I launch you into this rule, let's ask the most important question first: Does reading labels work—does it improve our health and slim our waist?

In a widespread review, the results of which were published in 2008, the U.S. Economic Research Service asked the same question. The answer was a clear yes. Compared to people who didn't read labels, label-readers consistently ate more fiber and thirteen other important dietary requirements necessary for better heart health and weight loss. Another study, this one of more than 3,700 men and women with heart problems, found that "those who read food labels consumed less energy, saturated fat, carbohydrates, and sugar, and more fiber than those who did not."

"Consuming less energy"—this is what we want!

And anyway, *that's what I said all along!*

Sorry for that outburst. But the fact is that using labels while you shop is getting easier. Not perfect, but a lot better. One reason for this improvement is that the government now requires clarity in food labeling. The other reason is more important: consumers—like you—are demanding it.

Following are the absolutely fundamental things to check when you read a label. The sooner you can store this information in your head, the more likely you'll be to buy the right foods to get and keep you slim. Remember the mantra: the more processed a food is, the more you should simply avoid it. Think of it as a boycott. Perhaps the only exception is frozen fruits and vegetables, which have been minimally processed. Fortunately you don't have to pay much attention to serving size for these because, for the most part, you can eat as much of them as you like.

Yes, I know you've been waiting for someone to say this for a long, long, time: an entire package of frozen spinach can be one serving!

Anyway, here are your marching orders—the pieces of information you need to look for on labels.

SERVING SIZE: It's right on the top, sometimes in bigger, bolder letters than the rest. Practice automatically scanning for this. Have some fun. Take your spouse/partner with you and play "guess the serving size." Pick up things all around the supermarket, from the deli to frozen food to canned items. Use your smartphone to find fun facts about the item. You'll see. Oh yeah, *you'll see* . . . something might look low-cal until you realize that a serving is about a tablespoon!

NUMBER OF SERVINGS: This is still the single most overlooked thing on the label. I can't tell you how many times I've had a client or contestant come up to me all excited about great "light" food, only to have me point out that what he thought was 250 calories is really 500 calories, because no one could possibly eat just half of what anyone would agree is a serving! But the knowledge helps them lose weight.

CALORIES: Once you've taken in the first two items, this is your first cut point. If the label says 350 calories per serving, and that means half of, say, a little protein bar that you'll eat in two bites, it's time to say goodbye. This is the first sign of a calorically dense food. You should be wary.

PROTEIN: With your daily requirement in mind (your weight divided by two equals the number of grams needed per day), this is one of the most important ingredients. If it's a low number, and you are looking for something to help fill your vital protein requirements, don't buy it.

SUGAR: By sugar, I mean sugars—all of them, from honey to agave to high fructose corn syrup. If it appears in the first five ingredients, keep walkin'.

SODIUM: Sodium is something we must have in our diets (see Rule 16). But not a lot. Unfortunately, many foods—including most prepackaged foods—have too much of it. The average American Jane or Joe scarfs down 3,300 mg of salt every day. The limit recommended for a healthy person is 2,400 mg. I say keep it under 2,000 mg.

FAT: Forget what you've been told. Fat is not a bad thing. Like salt, we need it. It's important that you get 25 to 35 percent of your daily calories from fat to keep you running. Back up near "serving size" you will find "calories of fat" per serving. Again, if you think you'd eat the whole thing, look back at the number of servings per package, then multiply the fat figure by that amount. You'll see just how much of your daily fat allotment you'll hog down when you eat that bag of trail mix. The label will also tell you the *percentage of fat calories per serving; if it is over 20 percent, walk away.* Also, remember that not all fats are equal. Look at the ingredients section to find out what kind of fat it is. If it is a saturated fat—lard, butter, oil, suet—it will be listed. Don't buy that product. Look for monounsaturated fats made from plants—olive oil, canola oil. For most weight losers, the daily quota is about 500 calories. Just for the record and in terms of those oils: That's. About. Five. Tablespoons.

TRANS FATS: The demon spawn of industrial food, trans fats are essentially highly saturated, inflammatory molecules used for convenience items likes cakes, donuts, cookies, and other baked items.

Trans fats help keep vending machine items fresh—for years. Do you really want that in your body? Unfortunately, trans fats do not have to be listed on the label if they weigh less than half a gram. That hidden trans fat can add up if you eat a lot of processed foods. Which is another great reason to stay away from processed foods and go to the ingredient source!

CARBS: As we've covered already, there are good carbs and bad carbs, refined versus unrefined. Check the ingredient list to see where the carbs come from. "Wheat flour?" No. "100 percent whole-wheat flour?" Yes. Potato starch. Uh-uh. Cornmeal, no—not if it's in the first five ingredients. Farro or barley? Yes. If you are diligent in this for a while, you'll develop your own go-to list of good carbs and thereby speed up the decision making when you shop.

FIBER: Remember, we are trying to get 30 to 50 grams a day. Paying attention to this number will really tell you something about how processed this item is. It will also give you a sense of how long this food will hang around in your gut. Also look in the ingredients section to see where this fiber comes from—whether it is added (OK in principle, as in the case of apple fiber or bran) or comes from industrial sources (not OK).

NET CARBS: This is where fiber pays off again! Net carbs are, in short, digestible carbs—the carbs that cause weight gain. The figure is arrived at by subtracting grams of fiber from total grams of carbohydrate. A piece of whole-wheat bread might weigh in at 25 grams of carbs, but when you take out 10 carbs of fiber, you've got 15 net carbs. I'll take fewer carbs any way I can get them. That said, check the ingredients to see where those carbs come from. If they come from processed grains, then no. If they come from whole grains, vegetables, and whole fruits—get it. If they're from "wheat flour," any added sugar, or anything you can't pronounce, skip it.

THE INGREDIENTS LIST: Usually located in microscopic type at the bottom of the label, this section tells you everything that goes into making the item. The top of the label tells you *how much* fat, for example, and this part of the label tells you *what kind* of fat. Ditto sugar—it could be any one of a number of sugars. One rule of thumb: the more items in this section, the less positively you should view this food. Why? For one, if it's got that many ingredients, it's probably incredibly processed—dense in chemicals that Mother Nature never intended you to eat. Two, it is dense in calories and low in fiber. In short: if a sweetener—any sweetener—or any refined flour (remember, it must say *whole*-wheat flour) appears within the first five ingredients, then just keep on pushing that grocery cart.

CHEMICALS: We live in a world of things like stabilizers, preservatives, and dyes, and escaping them entirely is unrealistic. (Unless you are wealthy, eccentric, or wealthy and eccentric.) But there are a few notorious ones, often found in diet and "lite" foods and you can avoid them if you know how to spot them:

Food dyes: Uncertainty about their health effects still reigns, but their prominence on the label tells you how fake the product in your hand is. Phony food—no!

Aspartame: The jury is still out about the connection between artificial sweeteners and various neurological conditions. I don't like the stuff—especially if it is in the top five ingredients. Why? Because aspartame, like high fructose corn syrup (HFCS) or lots of salt, keeps you in that appetite-twisting world of "hyperflavors," which have conditioned you to crave sugar, fat, and bad carbs.

Polysorbate 60: Pro-technology *Wired* magazine described polysorbate's main uses this way: "detergent, an emulsifier, or, in the case of polysorbate 60, a major ingredient in some sexual lubricants." There you go. Try not to eat it.

Olestra: Olestra products have labels. The labels say: "Olestra may cause abdominal cramping and loose stools. Olestra inhibits the absorption of some vitamins and other nutrients. Vitamins A, D, E, and K have been added." It can also cause diarrhea and anal leakage. Yay, Olestra!

MSG: A.k.a. monosodium glutamate, the stuff we know is in a lot of Chinese food. But packaged foods often come stuffed with it, the better to jack up our salt-craving taste buds. Many people are allergic to it: headaches, wheezing, nausea, difficulty breathing, tightness in the chest. Fun. If you are pregnant, do not eat anything with MSG in it.

Note: It is sometimes hard to spot MSG on the label because it has so many aliases. Among them are free glutamate, hydrolyzed proteins (any type), autolyzed yeast, yeast extract, caseinate, and "natural or artificial flavors."

Also note: MSG is also used for making "chewing gum, drinks, over-the-counter medications (especially children's), as a binder and filler for nutritional supplements, in prescription drugs, IV fluids given in hospitals, and in the chicken pox vaccine." As with Olestra, why would you want to *eat* this stuff?

THE "PERCENT OF DAILY VALUES" SECTION: This percentage comes courtesy of the standards for daily nutrition set by the FDA. Pay attention to how large a percentage of each nutritional component (calcium, sodium, vitamin C, and so on) a serving of this item will represent. As a general rule of thumb, if the percentage of daily values is less than 5 percent, it's not particularly nutritionally helpful. If it's got more than 20 percent of something—and as I say above about fat—walk away; that's too much. Although this information is written in annoyingly small type (and based on a 2,000-calorie-a-day diet, so factor that into your calculations), this section can be a great help once you've mastered the basics we've just gone through.

RULE 9

STOP GUESSING ABOUT
PORTION SIZE AND GET IT RIGHT—
FOR GOOD

How far out of whack are American portion sizes? Here is a story from a friend who wrote a book about obesity. A big hospital in Los Angeles was running a program for obese kids and their parents. Once a week, they would gather in one of the hospital's spacious conference rooms and review everything from exercise to food preparation. Instructors lined up a bunch of common food items on the front table and asked kids to show them what they considered to be a serving size. One item was a huge, family-sized bag of potato chips, clearly designed for use at a big picnic. A young girl was asked to show a portion size of it. "That's easy," she said, upon which she strode to the table, grabbed the entire bag, and walked back to her chair. "*That's* how much *I* eat!"

How did this happen? A lot of its boils down to the rise of

cheap foods and fats, which I cover in Rule 13. But some of it goes a little deeper, to something called portion distortion. In short, when people *see* large sizes, they *want* large sizes—at least a third more than they would normally eat. Studies show that this inclination has taken hold in American homes as well, with average at-home meals ballooning by 20 to 30 percent over the past twenty years. Amazingly, this desire for huge portions holds true even for *foods that are perceived as having a bad taste.* Like stale popcorn. That's a powerful force in your eating life. How can you fight it and win?

Making your own food (Rule 15) is one certain way. But for the moment, here are the two most basic tools I've got. They work for me, they work for clients, and they work for my team members on *The Biggest Loser.*

TECHNIQUE #1: FORCED PORTION CONTROL

If "forced portion control" sounds kind of bulimic to you, don't worry! It's most certainly not. By forced portion control, I mean buying, making, and being sure you've always got food that is ready to eat in the right amounts. (See my list of healthy, portion-controlled foods below.) No more "Oh, I slipped because I was famished by midafternoon and had only a quart of ice cream in the fridge." By the time you are done with this book, you'll always have a stash of delicious, fresh, and low-calorie foods in appropriate portions. Stuff you like. Sizes that make sense.

The bottom line: stock your kitchen with foods in portions you are sure about and/or portion it out into baggies or serving containers ahead of time so that when you're hungry, you find the right-sized offering.

MY FAVORITE FORCED PORTION-CONTROLLED FOODS

Plain Greek yogurt in 6-ounce containers

Individual low-fat cheese sticks

"Wholly Guacamole" individual servings of . . . guacamole

2-ounce bags of raw almonds

Pretty much every kind of fresh fruit, except *a whole darn watermelon!*

One tablespoon premeasured peanut butter packets

One hard-boiled egg

TECHNIQUE #2: HARPERSIZING

The second tool is what some have called "Harpersizing." It means that we take advantage of high-fiber, low-calorie foods that fill you up. We totally rethink their portion size. In fact, when it comes to vegetables and most fruits (see pages 105–7 for information on the best fruits to indulge in), you can forget portion size altogether. Eat what you want! I've been accused of going so far as to suggest that your Harpersized dinner could include a whole platter of broccoli.

Maybe that's an exaggeration for even the most broccoli-loving among us. But consider this: if you ate *half a pound* of fish with a huge serving of broccoli, along with half a cup of brown rice and an apple in Greek yogurt, you'd be eating about 590 calories, with lots of fiber, tons of protein, and no added fat or sugars. And you'd be full—that's a lot of food! (If you're on an 1,800-calorie regimen, you could eat two more meals *that day*!)

RULE 10

NO MORE ADDED SWEETENERS, INCLUDING ARTIFICIAL ONES

We are, as humans, hardwired to seek sweetness. It is a powerful, deeply rooted inclination. We even have specialized taste buds for it on our tongue. Think about it: in evolutionary terms, sweetness, as in berries and wild fruits, signaled something that was safe and edible and high in energy—what cavemen and -women needed to run all day.

We don't need to run all day.

That's why I want you to get away from *all* added sweeteners. Yes, I mean sweeteners in bread, sweeteners in frozen fruits (in the form of "added fruit concentrates"), and sweeteners in any packaged food you pick up on the fly. You don't have the physiological ammo to "just have a little." You don't have an antisweet taste bud. (You have a bitter one, but often even it acts in concert with the sweet bud.) I want you to get out of the whole world of hypersweetness. You won't psychologically expect supersweet when I'm done with you.

How critical is this step in terms of weight loss? After all, sugar is only 4 calories a gram; fat, which I have not eliminated altogether, is 9 calories. What's up with that?

In short, the 4 calories of sugar may have a more powerful weight-gain effect once they're in your body. By now I think you know you shouldn't go hog wild with high-fat cheeses, meats, or bacon. You should learn to think of sugars the same way—as a luxury. This represents a big change in thinking about sugar calories by the medical and nutritional big shots. For years, the American Heart Association fought the "sugar is just as destructive as fat" theory tooth and nail. They believed—and advocated along with the government—the low-fat gospel.

That changed with the obesity epidemic. Sixty percent of the population is now overweight, 30 percent of whom are obese. With that came the skyrocketing rates of type 2 diabetes. Health authorities and some controversial journalists began asking: if we have been on a low-fat diet binge for so long, why are we getting so porky?

The answer is sugar. Sugar and HFCS consumption soared, not just for the reasons we all know, but because even low-fat foods were chock full of it. And grains, especially refined grains, act much like sugar on the body's weight-control system. Sugar stimulates the liver to make new fat cells. And once you have a fat cell, you've got it forever.

Atkins-ism was one response, and it works—until you can't stand another steak-and-eggs breakfast sans toast. Then you go back to fatland. My way—and that of some others—tries to strike a balance between Atkins-ism and the low-fat doctrine. The Skinny Rules advocate using the *weight-lowering effects* of low-sugar/high-fiber fruits with the *satisfaction—or satiety—boost* we get from good fats. You're going to feel better and start losing pounds right from the start. And once you get used to that, you'll know why you can live without that soda!

Note: I am also asking you to banish artificial sweeteners like aspartame and stevia for the same basic reason—these sweeteners skew you to expect hypersweet tastes. If we don't get you out of that world, you'll keep expecting that reward. Believe me, this part of the step is worth the effort.

Does all this mean a life without dessert? No. In Rule 20, I'll tell you how to plan and successfully implement a weekly splurge meal. Trust me. There is a time and a place for cake, even in a rules life.

BE YOUR OWN SUGAR POLICE

What about sweeteners that *you* add—that teaspoon of brown sugar on your cereal, or that cube of sugar in your tea? What about the little blue packets of aspartame you automatically put in your coffee? Isn't that OK, since you can control the amount you use? My answer, as a trainer and as a weight-loss coach, is simple: no. But, as I have been trying to convince you, I have a heart as well as a brain. As is the case with diet soda, I'll give you a step-down option for this rule.

Enough with the added artificial sweeteners, OK? But if you can *really* stick to a teaspoon of brown sugar or a cube of sugar in your coffee or tea, step down from more of it this way: indulge yourself in that teaspoon or sugar cube NO MORE than twice a day. For your cereal? Add berries to sweeten things up.

RULE 11

GET RID OF THOSE WHITE
POTATOES

P op quiz: which food contributes more to weight gain over
any given period of time—soda, bacon and rich meats, or
baked potatoes?

The answer, according to our friends at the Nurses' Health
Study, is potatoes—in all forms, from fried to baked to roasted to
mashed: "For every additional daily serving of potatoes people ate,
they gained more than 1¼ pounds over a four-year period."

It's not that there is anything innately wrong with white potatoes; it's just that we consume so much of them, and in the most
overweight-producing forms. What's a lot? How about 125 pounds
a year, which at an average weight of 4–6 ounces each is about one
potato a day.

How do we do that? Tellingly, the National Institute of Diabetes
and Digestive and Kidney Diseases has the best data about potato
consumption: *Each year, Americans consume more than 4.5 billion
pounds of French fries (including more than two billion fast-food orders), snack on 6.7 billion pounds of potatoes processed into potato*

chips, and consume about 75 million pounds of Tater Tots. We like potatoes so much we're beginning to look like them.

And tragically, we eat them without the skin, where half the fiber and nutrients reside.

It says something that, if you're trying to eat the daily five servings of fruits and vegetables that all the experts recommend, you can't count potatoes, according to the U.S. Department of Agriculture (USDA). The benefits just don't outweigh the downside.

You know what's coming now.

You don't get to eat them anymore.

Or at least not like *that* anymore.

This is a pretty big change for many of us, and I was thinking perhaps I was being unreasonable by making this a rule. But then I looked around at the people who were most successful at losing weight and keeping it off. *None of them eat white potatoes in any form.* A formerly obese friend likes to say: "Bottom line, I abused my potato privileges!"

Fortunately, I can make this a little easier for you because nutrition science is showing that other tubers—like sweet potatoes (available in a golden yellow variety and in a deeper orange variety, which are often alternately labeled as yams in supermarkets), parsnips, turnips, and even many lesser-known kinds of potatoes—can earn a place on a weight-maintenance diet. (I still feel strongly, though, that even these should not be used in the first month of your regimen.) Yes, their preparation is a little more time consuming. But you're going to start treating starches as a kind of treat—remember? Potatoes in all forms are one of those starches. Moreover, there are weight-conscious ways to prepare root veggies that retain their fiber, which, as you know, cuts their net carbohydrate load. These methods are simple, easy, and tasty. And they enhance that sweet/savory character that I want you to nurture. We're leaving hypersalty, hyperfatty potatoes where they always belonged: in someone else's meal.

RAPID ROASTING: The best chefs in the world use this technique, as do some of the best home cooks I've ever met. Cut your sweet potatoes, turnips, or parsnips into one-inch cubes and spray them with olive or canola oil. Preheat the oven to 450°F, put them in on a baking sheet, and roast for about fifteen minutes. Take them out and sprinkle with pepper, minced garlic, lemon, or your favorite herbs. You can cook a bunch of these on Sunday night, let them cool, and place in the fridge. They will last all week, and you can use them in anything—soups, salads, even sandwiches, or as an accompaniment to your new repertoire of fish dishes!

FAKE FRYING: Fiber and taste are largely lost from root vegetables when you deep fry them. Keep the shape that reminds you of the deep-fried version, but "fake fry" those root vegetables and you'll retain the fiber and the taste, and you'll forego fat calories. This cooking technique is much like rapid roasting: take, say, some parsnips—those long, carrot-looking things next to the carrots at the market—and slice them lengthwise into fries. Toss them with some pepper and a tablespoon of olive oil. Get the oven up to 450°F, put the "fries" on a baking sheet, and let roast until they begin to brown.

WHOLE MASHING: You can kind of predict what this entails. You roast the root veggies (in addition to those described above, butternut squash and Jerusalem artichokes) *with the skin on* until they start to caramelize, let them cool, and then . . . mash (not blend). Because mashing concentrates calories, this is a perfect dish for your splurge meal (Rule 20), when you really want that mashed potato and gravy dish from back in the day.

RULE 12

MAKE ONE DAY A WEEK MEATLESS

More specifically, make one day a no-animal-protein day. Or go meatless/animal-protein-less more than one day if you want. The more the better.

Why do I want you to do this?

One reason, and one reason only: it will help you lose weight and keep it off.

And if you learn to use a few simple plant foods well, it will keep you from succumbing to that notorious dieter's trap: monotony.

Doubt this?

Trust my process.

A meatless day can still provide you with an abundance of fruits and Harpersized platters of vegetables. You know by now that I want you to get a lot of protein, a lot of fiber, as few simple sugars as possible, and no bad fats.

What other foods meet this criteria? Answer: beans and nuts or seeds.

Both of these food groups tend to be underused in our daily American diet. Nuts are relegated to snack time. Nut butters to children. And beans? My bet is you almost never eat them, unless they're made with huge amounts of added fat and sugar.

The common excuse, especially for beans, is that they are inconvenient to cook and taste rather bland. They also give you gas. I'd disagree with the first two statements and the third is not as pronounced as the kids' rhyme about beans would make it seem!

Beans are technically the fruit of a family of plants called the Leguminosae. They are high in protein—the tiny green lentil, for example, gets one-fourth of its calories from protein—as well as low in fat and high in fiber. A single cooked half-cup serving gives you 9 grams of fiber; subtract that from 20 grams of carbs and you've got a tasty 11-carb, 110-calorie dish that has one of the highest concentrations of plant protein you can get. And almost no fat. That's a combination that will leave you satisfied and, eventually, slimmer. No wonder *Men's Health* magazine named lentils as one of the five healthiest foods to be had.

Two other beans worth knowing about are garbanzo and white beans. Both are commonly used throughout the world and increasingly so in urban areas of the United States with big ethnic populations. The garbanzo is inexpensive and, perhaps best of all, easily available in both dry and canned form. The canned form is an easy way to get 9 grams of fiber per serving; dried beans are less expensive but require an overnight soak. The same can be said for white beans. As the recipe section will show, these beans are incredibly versatile and tasty. If you weren't a bean person before, you will be soon.

Nuts are also tree fruits, and they have been critical parts of the human diet since recorded history. Nuts—almonds, walnuts, and pistachios—are pretty much ideal foods so long as you eat them raw or dry-roasted (stay away from salted or honey-roasted and those salty "mixed nut" jars!). They are high in protein, fiber, good fats, and those beneficial phytochemicals we discussed in Rule 6.

But nuts have gotten a bad rap. They are mainly seen as high-fat snack foods to be avoided when people want to lose weight. I think this comes from the same seventies and eighties thinking that had us obsess about fats rather than carbohydrates. Peanut butter was once singled out as a "heart attack food" right along with fast-food burgers.

Yet for almost two decades, nutritional science—especially that concerned with obesity and heart disease—has tacked back in favor of nuts. As early as 1991 big studies were reporting a strong link between eating daily portions of nuts and low rates of heart disease. If you take a blood sample from a dieter eating nuts versus one not eating nuts, you'll see a lot more good cholesterol, a lot less bad cholesterol, and a big decrease in something called C-reactive protein, an inflammatory molecule that can cause heart attack and stroke.

What about our main concern in the rules—weight loss? Nuts look good there, too.

A recent experiment by UCLA's Center on Human Nutrition looked at a group of obese people with BMIs of 31, just over the defining cutoff point of 30 for obesity. (That's where a lot of us are—just fat enough to get into health trouble.) Both groups were put on the same diet, with one difference. One group ate 240 calories of pretzels while the other ate 240 calories of pistachios. Both groups lost weight, but the pistachio effect was so strong as to drive BMI down to 28—no longer obese. The pretzel group lost almost no body mass.

How could that be? You guessed it: some foods cause weight loss more than others, even if their calories are the same. In the case of nuts, the effect seems to come from two mechanisms. They are important to remember because my Skinny Rules are constantly seeking to use and exploit these mechanisms.

The first is the one we already know about—fat causes satiety, and that makes you eat less. But there is also another tool in nuts' weight-loss arsenal. Eating them seems to briefly—but significantly—raise your resting energy expenditure, or REE. In a study of nut consumption during a diet, Purdue University scholars recorded substantial increases in sedentary calorie burning in dieting patients who ate nuts versus dieters who did not. This led them to proclaim: "The few trials contrasting weight loss through regimens that include or exclude nuts indicate improved compliance and greater weight loss when nuts are permitted. This consistent literature suggests nuts may be included in the diet, in moderation, to enhance palatability and nutrient quality without posing a threat for weight gain."

Again, that's what I said!

As you get into the menus in Part II, you'll see just how much I like beans and nuts. If you come over to my place during midafternoon, you might find me resting my energy expenditure out on my patio, eating one of my favorite new snacks, hummus (made mostly of garbanzo beans) with cucumber slices and a squeeze of lemon. The combination tastes great, and you'll end up getting as much as a quarter of your daily fiber when you eat it.

The same with nut butters. Often I have one slice of toasted Ezekiel bread (80 calories), one tablespoon of peanut butter (100), and half a banana (40) for an afternoon snack. As you'll see in the menus in Part II, nut butter snacks fit into our rules easily and effectively. It's time to get nuts. And beans!

RULE 13

GET RID OF FAST FOODS
AND FRIED FOODS

For many modern eaters, it's hard to imagine a time when fast foods—from TV dinners to double cheeseburgers—were a rare treat, but they were. Two generations ago they were costly and sometimes hard to find (there were far fewer fast-food "restaurants" on the face of the planet). Portions were smaller. Think of those tiny TV dinners of the 1960s and 1970s, the ones that scalded your (or your parents') tongue with those little hot apple pie portions. We also did not have places like the Cheesecake Factory where, whether you dine in or take out, you can consume the entire caloric requirements for an entire village at one sitting.

But that is how it was—fast-food scarcity!—until three things happened:

1. The government encouraged overplanting of crops like corn and soy (to sell to global markets).

2. Food companies used low-priced corn to make less expensive sugars, allowing them to sell supersized portions cheaply.

3. A new-style American family emerged, with two parents working and no time to cook.

Earl Butz, the head of the USDA in the 1970s, hit the lure of premade food right on the head: "TV dinners and fast foods are built-in maid service!"

OK, there's something positive to be said for a food system that adapts quickly to changing needs. But when eating fast, preprocessed, and jumbo becomes a default behavior, you've got problems. In essence, you simply lose control over your diet. Restaurant portions are usually 40 to 50 percent bigger than what you'd serve at home, and because even daily dining out is still viewed as a "treat" by most people, they eat like it's a birthday celebration for Uncle Joe. The more they eat out, the more they overeat. (See Rule 15 for more on the benefits of eating at home!)

Even *standing* inside a fast-food restaurant reinforces the problem. Your powerful sense of smell gets hijacked by all those high-fat molecules filling up the air around you. You also lose control of your sense of taste. Soon, anything that is not hypersweet or salty falls short of your desire and just doesn't do it for you. You're a prisoner of fast food. Not an addict. A prisoner.

That will change with this diet. By the time I am done with you, you'll want to run the other way when you smell fast food.

Now, what happens, exactly, when you eat jumbo whipped cheddar mashed potato nuggets? Or a bag of French fries? Or a slice of double-stuffed deep-dish pizza with sausage and pepperoni?

Let's start with what happens when it goes into your mouth. Here we begin the long and expensive and ugly slide to a mouth full of cavities and various tooth diseases. Concentrated fats and sugars also stimulate strong inflammatory reactions by your body's immune system. Often that reaction begins in the esophagus. There is actually an emergency medical condition called "steakhouse syndrome" in which the huge shot of bad fats into the bloodstream that occurs after ingestion of high-fat meats results in cardiac distress. Make no mistake, you have to leave the steakhouse and go to the ER for that.

But let's say you avoided the ER and now the fries and burger are in your gut. For starters, there's a good chance you'll be tasting it all day and maybe all night; fried foods can cause heartburn and esophageal reflux. In your bloodstream, bad cholesterol soars. If you've got a heart condition already, you are in danger—and I am not exaggerating. Heart attacks and strokes soar within the first two to three hours of such meals. The connection is so strong that, when the University of Michigan studied neighborhoods with lots of fast-food joints, it found the risk of stroke in a neighborhood increased by 1 percent for every fast-food restaurant.

Let us now come to your pancreas and liver. Chronic eating of concentrated sugars and bad fats tells the organs to make more insulin and more blood fat, as your muscles become resistant to the insulin. This is called type 2 diabetes. It's not benign. Too much insulin floats around your bloodstream and destroys nerves. If you get a cut, it takes longer to heal. If you don't start taking meds, you can eventually lose your eyesight.

Yet for many of us, all this medical stuff doesn't matter. What matters is, as Billy Crystal used to say on *Saturday Night Live* (paraphrasing Fernando Lamas), "It's not how you feel, it's *how you look!*" And if you keep eating the way you have been, you aren't going to look so great. There's the obvious rotundity and the accompanying social stigma. Also, chronic consumption of fast food will prematurely age your skin. I am not exaggerating. If you review the work of legitimate skin researchers, you find a litany of

fat- and sugar-fueled rashes, accelerated wrinkling, eyelid droop-
ing, and muscle shrinking.

But we are not done. Stay with me. If you keep going down the
fast-food path, you may get a bad case of sleep apnea—the extra
weight can push down on your throat while you sleep and cut off
air flow. That will make you sleepy and sluggish all day. Soon you'll
be put on what's called a C-pap machine, which requires you to
wear a plastic mouthpiece while you sleep. It inevitably causes a
rash of whiteheads and blackheads, not to mention that it doesn't
look very sexy in bed!

Is there any way to eat fast foods (a.k.a. highly processed, likely
fried) or fried foods and be healthy? No.

A FAT WARNING SIGN FOR YOUR REFRIGERATOR DOOR

What are the main side effects of eating fried foods? Post this list on
your refrigerator door to remind yourself why you should stay away
from them:

Eating fried foods can cause . . .

- GERD (gastroesophageal reflux disease)
- chronic diarrhea
- "anal leakage" (not kidding)
- acne, skin rashes, and cholesterol "bumps" under eyes
- halitosis and smelly skin
- high bad cholesterol and low good cholesterol
- irritable bowel syndrome
- gallstones

Need I say more?

RULE 14

EAT A REAL BREAKFAST

I f you're like me you probably put this age-old advice in the same file with such commands as "eat your spinach," "take out the trash," or "get off the couch and stop playing video games."

You kinda ignore it.

Don't. I'm not telling you to eat breakfast because it is "healthy," I'm telling you that *you will fail at weight loss and weight control if you don't.*

Why? Because my experience tells me it's essential. If there is one habit all my contestants on *TBL* have in common, it's skipping breakfast.

And if that isn't proof enough for you, you should take note that, over and over, researchers find that people who skip breakfast are more likely to eat too many calories later in the day—calories that come from bad foods. Consider:

From the University of Massachusetts Medical School: "Breakfast skippers are 4.5 times more likely to be obese than are breakfast eaters. That may be partly because breakfast skippers tend to make up the calories throughout the day with less healthy alternatives, and also because breakfast eaters are also giving their metabolism a boost."

From the journal *Pediatrics:* "Breakfast eaters often had a higher daily caloric intake and yet also a lower BMI than their breakfast-skipping peers . . . [but there were] inverse associations between breakfast frequency and BMI." Translation: the more often you skip breakfast, the more likely you are to be overweight.

From the *European Journal of Neuroscience:* "Skipping breakfast . . . increased the activation [of brain reward centers] to pictures of high-calorie over low-calorie foods in the [brain] . . . and enhanced the appeal of high-calorie more than low-calorie foods." Translation: skipping breakfast will make you want bad foods more than good foods later in the day. Not good.

Do I have your attention?

When should you eat breakfast? I prefer that you eat it within an hour of waking and, of course, *after a large glass of water.* I don't have a bushel of studies about this, but I do have a lot of experience as a personal trainer of people with weight problems. And to a person, this is often the hardest change they must make. Dieters tend to believe that the fewer meals they eat, the more likely they will lose weight. That's a tough habit to break.

Break it.

I offer some delicious breakfast menus in Part II, but for now, here are three key foods to have for breakfast:

OATMEAL: Oatmeal, along with all of its heart-healthy attributes, also helps you lose weight—it's one of those Nurses' Health Study foods we talked about. When you compare eating calorie-matched oatmeal versus other cereals, you're more likely to reduce your waistline. You'll get better control over your blood sugar and insulin, so you'll feel less hungry. You'll get fiber (4 grams), only 21 net carbs, almost no fat (unless *you put it in*), and only 150 calories. Whether you prepare steel-cut oatmeal or go for the convenience of a just-add-hot-water instant packet (no sweetened ones, sorry), you're doing yourself a huge and filling favor! Add half a cup of blueberries (or raspberries or blackberries—remember, berries are your friends!) if you want, a little skim milk, and you're at 200. Not enough for you? Then consider the oatmeal your breakfast warm-up and keep going with a next breakfast course of . . .

EGGS: The nutritional bad boy of the eighties and nineties, eggs have emerged as a prized element of a healthy, weight-conscious diet. They're low in calories, high in protein, and have zero carbs; in the case of egg whites there is *no* fat and only *20 calories apiece.* You can have a five-white omelet with one (preferably omega-3) yolk thrown in for taste and color, and you've got a 140-calorie protein bomb. Now add all the veggies you want—mushrooms, tomatoes, spinach—and you're at 200 calories. With the oatmeal, 350. Add a tablespoon of ricotta cheese, and you are at 400. What a way to start the day!

GREEK YOGURT: This is the closest thing I have to a magic ingredient. It's my version of the *French Women Don't Get Fat* leek broth, if you will. Except it's Greek. And white. And tasty.

Now that I think of it, it has no resemblance at all to leek broth! But its weight-loss properties do.

Greek yogurt, now available under many brand names, gets my applause for a bunch of reasons. Guess which is first? That's right. It tastes good. It can be used for just about anything, from dessert (with fruit, nuts, etc.) to breakfast (with berries, or as a warm-up to your eggs, as explained above), for dinner (add herbs or spices or mustard and you've got a sauce for some fish and meats), or for a midday snack. Greek yogurt is thicker than regular yogurt; it gives you that great ice cream mouthfeel. It's got lots of healthy bacteria. But your reason for eating a lot of it is simple: it increases your feeling of satisfaction after a meal. Much more than, say, fruit juices or fruit-dairy smoothies. Greek yogurt now comes in all kinds of fruit-added, no-fat flavors, but go for the plain variety and doctor it up yourself with berries and nuts. Remember, we're trying to kick the sweet taste habit!

WAKE UP AND DO THESE THINGS!

- Be prepared: if you know your morning will be rushed, make sure you've got lots of individualized proteins (yogurt cups or hard-boiled eggs), a grain (an oatmeal packet), and some berries in a plastic container. You don't get a pass from the rules just because you're busy.
- Prep your fiber fruit: cut up the apple the night before and put the slices in an airtight container or sealed plastic bag.
- Protein, protein, protein: get up and eat your eggs or yogurt.
- Oatmeal, oatmeal, oatmeal: get up and pop that packet into the microwave.
- Water, water water: fill the glass and put it on your bedside table the night before. Not kidding. Do it.

RULE 15

———

MAKE YOUR OWN FOOD
AND EAT AT LEAST TEN MEALS
A WEEK AT HOME

H ow do you call your family to dinner? Is it by saying, "OK you kids, *get in that car!*"

If so, that's going to change. You've got to cook.

I know, I know. Is Harper crazy? Doesn't he know how busy I am?

Too bad! Harper's Way is not easy. I told you that when we started. The old easy way got you here! If you want to change your life, and not just your lifestyle, you've got to do things differently. Or stay fat. Period.

I can't emphasize this rule enough. I eat at home and cook for myself as often as I can, and my contestants on the show cook for themselves, too. And remember, some of them were eating *all* their meals out before they came on the show. If they can make the change, so can you.

Cooking and eating at home at least ten times a week (which is really only one meal at home a day, and more on just a few more days) is the next logical step for those of you who've already given up fast food. (Congratulations!) But this does not mean you've got to buy all kinds of fancy gadgets, or start reading Julia Child and watching cooking shows every night. It requires only a little planning, a willingness to learn some basics, and some creativity on your part to make your food something you and others in your family look forward to eating.

Just planning your meals makes a huge impact on weight loss. When scholars writing in the journal *Appetite* studied hundreds of dieters, they found that those who reported planning meals were more than twice as likely to lose weight. Ditto a series of studies from our friends at Harvard.

I'll take those odds.

Of course, for many families, this step will incite a domestic culture clash between the "eating alone on the run" way and the "dinner will be served at 6:30" way. Each of you will negotiate this in your own fashion. Maybe you'll cook healthy, rule-abiding foods and portion them out in containers in the fridge so that everyone can grab and go at their convenience. Remember, you're not going to even *have* certain foods in the house anymore—so not only will you not stock chips, sodas, mac and cheese, and sugary cereals as options for the others, you'll eventually be able to live without the whining for those kinds of foods (if you stick to your guns and follow the rules). Maybe you'll try to institute some new rules of your own about the timing and attendance of family meals. Whatever you do, the key is to eat more of the food that you cook yourself, that you control, and that you can trust.

WHY—REALLY—THE FRENCH AREN'T FAT

We can take some guidance from that fashionably slender people on the other side of the Atlantic: the French. It was the French, back in the early part of the twentieth century, who created the modern way of table-dining. And I am not talking about sitting around for a four-hour meal. Rather, I mean the daily meal rules:

- Do not put large platters of food on the table. When you put second portions in front of you, you're more likely to eat like it's Thanksgiving rather than, say, Gandhi's birthday.
- If possible, do not eat alone. Eat as a couple, or as a family.
- Do not eat away from the table. The table is where you eat. Even when you snack. The couch is where you watch TV, read this book, or meditate.
- Set the table—even if this means the most rudimentary plate, napkin, fork, and glass on a placemat. After all, the table is where you eat, not *feed*.
- Allow no distractions at the table. Especially no TV.

CHANGES WHEN SHOPPING

Your first real change will be when you go shopping. The basics are intuitive. In the spirit of planning ahead, make a shopping list. Put question marks next to the items you don't know enough about—salt content, organic or no, and so forth. Take a pen to check things off or make notes. If there is a meat counter or butcher, ask about special cuts of meats or fish and purchase only the amount you need (those precut shrink-wrapped meats are often for families of four, so avoid them unless you need that much). Butchers are so used to being ignored they'll love the attention. This is your life—make your own food world or be at the mercy of others.

Check your shopping pattern: are most of the items coming from the periphery, where you find produce, proteins, and fiber, or from the aisles, where most preprocessed foods reside? Strive to stay along the walls of the store! This may be the single most important piece of advice from the person I consider to be the nation's best food writer, Michael Pollan. By doing so, you'll not only buy the right foods, but you'll also send a signal to the store manager to pay more attention to whole, healthy, unprocessed products.

CHANGES AT HOME

In Part II I'll give you a number of ideas for setting yourself up for success, but for the moment, do yourself this favor: put the least caloric and most rule-abiding things at eye level in the fridge and pantry.

Next, get your kitchen ready. First, take a quick inventory of your kitchen tools. There are some basics: a blender, a toaster, a nice big skillet, a large pot for boiling water, a big roasting pan, a decent knife set, a couple of plastic cutting boards of different sizes, an immersion blender (a.k.a. stick blender). Invest in a slow cooker. Get a couple of clear vinegar and oil bottles. Buy a bunch of sealable plastic bags and containers of different sizes so you can pre-portion-control meals and snacks.

Next: get a good reference book that lists the calories, fiber, fat, and carbs of all common foods. A good one is *The CalorieKing Calorie, Fat and Carbohydrate Counter* by Allan Borushek. Use this book! Really read it, paying attention also to serving size and salt content.

What about your dry pantry? Stock up on all your basic spices and dried herbs, making sure you've got whole peppercorns for your pepper mill, cinnamon, and vanilla and that your oregano isn't five years old (better yet, get some fresh oregano and other herbs since you'll be using them in your Skinny cooking). Throw away that dusty tin of garlic flakes and buy some fresh garlic bulbs. You should have olive oil, tuna fish, canned tomatoes, garbanzo beans, hummus, and low-salt chicken stock. Order a box of single-portion peanut butter and guacamole packets. Get some high-bran crackers like GG Bran Crispbread.

Also: buy bags of single-portion frozen brown rice plus farro, quinoa, lentils, barley, and oatmeal. Get some of those individual microwavable packets of oatmeal as well. Stock a bunch of good whole-wheat pasta. Check the label. You now know what to check. Throw away all white-grain products.

A few things should always be in your refrigerator: plain Greek yogurt in single-serving containers, apples, berries, string cheese, ricotta or cottage cheese, grated parmesan cheese, Ezekiel bread, a half pound of cheddar or Swiss cheese, a quart of low- or no-fat milk, and some fresh green beans and cucumbers (Persian are my favorites) for snacking. And some lemons, since a squirt of their juice can help you kick your salt habit. Lemon brings out the flavor in all kinds of foods.

MY SODA ELIMINATOR

Remember, your aim is to stop drinking soda. Not only full-calorie soda, but the diet stuff as well. So, what to drink? I use a simple appliance made by SodaStream that turns regular water into soda water. Often I then squeeze into it some lemon or lime, and I've got my own soda. It's nice to have with your midafternoon snack, and it staunches some of your craving for something sweet to go with something savory.

RULE 16

BANISH HIGH-SALT FOODS

I f there is a common source of anxiety among my trainees and *Biggest Loser* contestants, it's got to be salt. They are eager to learn how much they consume. They are anxious at the idea of eating less. As is the case with too many Americans, they eat too much of it. Way too much. The Mayo Clinic tells us that the average person should get no more than 2,300 milligrams of sodium a day, about a teaspoon. The average American consumes 3,400. The average *TBL* contestant? I've seen folks who routinely eat 5,000 or 6,000 milligrams a day! Most of these earnest dieters are shocked when they learn that, and I'll bet you would be too if you calculated how much salt you ingest every day.

Why is salt so vexing? Because we are often misled about it. It is common to see a label claiming that a product is "low salt," "heart healthy," or "low sodium," and indeed it is—if you eat the tiny recommended portion (twelve potato chips?!). Also, salt is the most common added ingredient in all processed foods, from applesauce to tuna fish to tomato soup to peanut butter. Figuring it out is often neither simple nor intuitive. When you put canned carrots, for instance, in your cart, you are probably trying to do the right thing—there are veggies in that can, after all. But take a closer look: 230 milligrams of salt per serving. (Fresh carrots, by contrast, have 40 milligrams per serving.)

The food industry is at its absolute worst when it comes to salt and salt labeling. Between the colorful labels, tiny and confusing type, and bad recipe recommendations, the issue is not so straightforward. They don't make it easy, and you've got to take control.

Here's more: our bodies *need* salt to remain in chemical balance, but each individual's requirements can fluctuate wildly. When a couch potato becomes physically active, he needs more salt. It's not just a matter of cutting it out completely.

It gets complicated.

But it needn't be. The simple rule of thumb is that you need to eat less than 2,000 milligrams of salt a day. Think about that number when you reach for salt or when you're considering something salty. Limit yourself to that number or less.

For the overweight and obese, salt commands attention for two reasons. The first is health. Too much salt and you will upset your body's exquisite mechanism for maintaining proper levels of fluid. That causes increased blood volume, which makes your heart work harder to move blood through arteries, which increases blood pressure. Like anything under too much pressure, something's going to blow. When it does, we call it stroke or heart disease. It is a leading cause of premature death in the general population. It is *the* leading cause of premature death among women.

There are less grave but nonetheless important consequences as well; swollen "Cabbage Patch doll" ankles, dry skin, and puffy bags under the eyes. Fluid retention also can slow weight loss and cause you to get discouraged. You don't need that.

Once dieters get their salt basics under control, they get creative. As one *TBL* contestant reported on my blog, "I used to add salt to everything because my mom did . . . I found that I could add pepper and basil with a couple other herbs and still get a great tasting chicken, fish, etc. Cooking w/ lemon and other citrus helps add extra flavor also. I've started using saltless butter when I use butter so that I can add salt to taste and not already have salt added."

Here's how I manage my salt intake:

- Don't use salt at the table. Don't even put it on the table; having it there will make it too easy to add to your food without thinking. If you really think something needs salt, you'll have to get up to get the shaker. That's a disincentive right there.
- When you check a label for salt content, always check portion size as well.
- Use lemons and lemon juice to enhance flavors.
- If something you're cooking calls for a teaspoon of salt, start with a half or a third instead. You can always add more later. You can't take it out.

RULE 17

EAT YOUR VEGETABLES— JUST DO IT!

Let's just acknowledge from the beginning that we've all been hearing this refrain since we were able to throw a temper tantrum at the dinner table.

The advice didn't stick.

It felt like a punishment. Veggies were tasteless and mushy and made you think "hospital."

Or "cafeteria."

Or "prison."

They smelled funny.

Adults seemed obsessed with getting you to eat them.

And, let's face it: "It's good for you" just does not work. We know it's good for us and we *just don't care!*

But what if I told you that if you *added* some tasty, crisp, and easy-to-prepare veggies to your daily diet that you would feel more satisfied, naturally eat less, and *lose* weight?

Doing so works for me—and it works for my clients. I see it

over and over again. The same guys who told me that vegetables are "a hassle" are now coming back to me with creative recipes for their newfound favorite vegetable! Weight loss and great taste: how did that strange combination happen?

You can figure out part of the answer. Vegetables have a huge amount of fiber, which, shall we say, makes the trains run on time. They consist principally of water. They have few sugars and few calories.

OK, so what's new? Just how powerful are these forces? One of our era's great nutrition scientists, Penn State's Barbara Rolls, has been exploring that issue for almost two decades now. Mainly interested in childhood obesity, Rolls has long understood the complexity of eating choices and weight management. With the benefit of experience, she's learned something that might sound strange: you've got to trick the body into eating less, and veggies may be the most powerful way to do this. Over the years she has found ways to "sneak" veggies into children's meals; the kids end up eating less of the calorie-rich foods. She's secretly introduced veggie purees into regular dishes—and found that eaters routinely eat less all day long.

That's why vegetable soup—don't worry; I've got easy ways to make it taste *amazing*—will be one of your biggest friends. You'll want more. As Rolls puts it in her no-nonsense style: "When soup was consumed [15 minutes before the main meal], subjects reduced meal energy intake by 20%."

I'll take that.

Rolls has found the same effect with raw veggies, leafy veggies, and veggie purees.

You'll find a list of all-you-can eat veggies on pages 103–4 (as well as a shorter list of vegetables you should go easy on), but first let me talk about two that have particularly great taste and versatility.

The first is **kale.** You see kale, a long-overlooked green, on all the healthy-eating lists lately. And for good reason. It's loaded with vitamins C and K, calcium, and fiber. Along with broccoli, a sister crop (see below), it's recently become the object of interest of researchers studying ways to counteract chronic inflammation, the key instigator of many modern diseases as well as aging. Scientists at Johns Hopkins single out kale and broccoli for their high quantities of a chemical called sulforaphane. UCLA scientists have shown that sulforaphane may someday be used to reduce the toxic effects of smog on the respiratory system.

That's great—but what about our main concern, weight loss? Kale has no magical effects; it just fits so perfectly in our new eating pattern. To wit: a huge, "Harperian" portion of kale (an entire bunch from the store) is only 50 calories. It's easy to prepare—and like spinach and any number of green leafies, the frozen version retains all of its nutritional benefits. You can stir-fry it, steam it, put it in soups. Perhaps just as important: it tastes great. Kale, along with a number of other veggies listed here, will diversify your diet and get you plugged into a new world of slimming foods with enticing new tastes. Slowly but surely, it will replace your unhealthy world of supersweet and supersalty.

Broccoli, in all its forms, is my other super-weight-loss vegetable. I say "in all its forms," because too often when we say broccoli we *see* in our minds that dreaded junior high cafeteria line, with its smelly vats of mushy, tasteless florets.

But it does not have to be that way. I'll get to some recipes later, but I want you to do two things now. First, go to your supermarket and look for broccoli rabe—the tangy Italian green often sold as rapini—or Broccolini, a fairly new hybrid that usually comes in small spears ready to cook. If they don't carry either ask the produce guy to order them. Now go home, boil a big pot of water, and plunge in one of these alternative broccolis. (You will have to break apart and peel the stalks of the rapini, but stop complaining and just do it!) Take it out in two minutes, drain, and add some lemon juice mixed with a tablespoon of olive oil. Eat. Enjoy.

You've now mastered one of your most important new cooking techniques—one that will go a long way toward making you slimmer, fitter, and happier.

THE POWER OF SOUP

There was a time when soup occupied a much more central role in the American diet. It was inexpensive, filling, full of nutrients—and easy to make. But it took a little time, both to make (chop chop chop) and to eat. You could not eat soup out of one hand on the freeway. But for the weight-loser like yourself, soup remains a key tool for good nutrition and feeling full. Over and over, scholars who examine eating patterns find the same thing: people who consume soups regularly tend to feel fuller longer, and thus tend to eat less. And, really, how hard are they to make, especially these days, when low- and no-salt broths are on the shelves of supermarkets everywhere? I've got a few basic recipes in Part III. If you do yourself a favor and start making soup by my Skinny Rules, you're going to come up with gobs of recipes on your own.

RULE 18

_____

GO TO BED HUNGRY

Why is this so hard? I have a couple ideas, one based on research and experience, one based on armchair psychology.

In the physical realm, you know what happens when you haven't eaten: your stomach feels empty, maybe a little achy, in need of comfort. You crave carbs. And yes, carbs can make you feel better in the short term. But as you now know, that benefit soon turns into a hunger-producing monster. In the psychological realm, overweight people are often lonely and anxious; eating before bed is nerve-settling, comforting.

Given these obstacles, is bedtime fasting worth it? Absolutely. Because you will burn fat like crazy if you do it. The absence of carbs in your bloodstream will let your body produce the hormones it needs for better sleep. And with good sleep comes other benefits—muscle repair, brain-chemical balancing, and increased energy during the day. You might almost say that sleep is nature's ultimate spa treatment. It's no accident that the connection between sleep and obesity is one of the hottest scientific enterprises going. Which leads us to Rule 19 (see page 86).

HOW TO MAKE YOURSELF COMPLY

There are a lot of ways one might comply with this rule: Don't eat three hours before going to bed. Don't eat after eight. Don't eat anything after dinner. You decide. Your body will respond: denied fuel for more than five hours, your body will start burning its own fat and sugar. That means that, if your dinner was at 8 p.m., you're burning fat by 1 a.m.

AMUSING THINGS TO DO AT NIGHT INSTEAD OF EATING

Men
- Watch *Die Hard* again . . . and again, and again. You can never go wrong with *Die Hard*.
- Find your old high school girlfriend on Facebook and "poke" her.
- Read the instruction manual on that new camera of yours. . . . I'm sure you will learn a lot more than just point and shoot.
- Search travel websites for your next big bachelor party in Vegas. Remember, what happens in Vegas, etc.
- Take all your "fat clothes," box them, and label it FAT CLOTHES

Women
- Watch *Steel Magnolias* again. . . . Don't forget the Kleenex.
- Find your best friend from high school on Facebook and re-kindle that friendship.
- Read the instruction manual on your new smartphone and re-alize all the really cool things that you are missing out on when it comes to what they can do now.

- Search travel websites for your next big girls' weekend/spa get-away in VEGAS!!! (Same rules from above apply.)
- Ditto, then go out and buy an entire new wardrobe for that Vegas spa weekend.

If going to bed hungry sounds tough to you, start small. For the first month, try going to bed hungry one night a week. No more. Plan for it by marking it on your calendar. Put a sign on your refrigerator door reminding you to:

1. Ask yourself what you really want before you open that door (sleep? company? reassurance that everything will be all right?).
2. Think: "I can eat tomorrow night."

Set up a reward system for compliance. If you succeed one night, promise yourself a massage, a movie, even a new pair of shoes.

Yes, a *new pair of shoes. That's* it!

RULE 19

SLEEP RIGHT

You don't have to go to any textbook to be told that you should get eight hours of sleep a night. When you sleep, your body heals. When you sleep, all that work we do in the gym slowly turns into muscle. Sleep gives your various overactive brain synapses a chance to reoxygenate and settle down. That's why you feel so refreshed after a good sleep.

But I also like to think of sleep just the way you would anything else in this list of rules: as an ingredient in your weight-loss diet. It's just as important as protein, fiber, whole grains, and fat.

Easier said than done.

Because it really doesn't matter whether you are overweight or not: sleep gets harder the older you get. That's mainly because your body stops making the hormones critical for sound sleep. Add to this the overstimulation of modern life, and you've got a recipe for an epidemic of sleeplessness. Some experts estimate that 20 percent of Americans don't get nearly enough sleep. And so far, the pharmaceutical industry has some work to do to make an effective drug to help. Sleep has turned out to be as vexing as it is important. I still struggle with it.

The overweight and obese have other huge issues with sleep. If you are obese, you will likely, at some point, become an apneac—your excess weight can cut off your air flow, causing heavy snoring and restricted breathing. At best, this will leave you chronically fatigued during the day. At worst, sleep apnea poses a severe risk of heart attack.

The more disturbed your sleep pattern, according to a recent study from the University of Chicago, the more likely you are to lose control of your eating the next day: "Alterations in the balance between sleep and wakefulness can modify the amount, composition, and distribution of human food intake and suggest that sleeping short hours in modern societies may aggravate the problem of excessive energy consumption."

The upshot: you'll snack on high-calorie foods. And you'll get fat.

Men should pay particular attention to sleep. Studies show that sleep deprivation makes them *more* vulnerable to snacking and weight gain than women. This is a phenomenon my writing partner's wife calls "the only social justice ever conferred upon dieting women." I agree.

HOW TO GET SOME SHUT-EYE

No one knows exactly how to make someone sleep better, but let me give you some general rules that seem to work for me:

1. Avoid alcohol after eight. Because alcohol is a depressant, you'd think it would make you sleep better. But anyone who's ever drunk too much booze too late in the day knows that isn't the case. Alcohol is just another form of sugar, and sugar destabilizes the low metabolic state needed to sustain sleep.
2. Avoid coffee, tea, and other stimulants after 3 p.m. This is because stimulants . . . stimulate.
3. Talk to your physician about the pros and cons of sleeping aids and sleeping medication. I don't mean to sound like one of those prescription drug commercials you see on TV, but I want to impress on you that (a) while I have no fundamental problem with your using all the sleep-promoting tools at your disposal, (b) I *do* want you to be an active player in that decision. Educate yourself about sleep. Check out the University of Maryland's Sleep Disorders Institute site at www.umm.edu/sleep/adult_sleep_dis.htm.
4. If you must eat: eat vegetables and high-fiber fruits. Also, chamomile or valerian root tea.
5. Make your own sleep spa: Use some aromatic soaps in your bathwater. Get a white-noise machine. Put a dab of lavender oil on each temple and below your nose.
6. Unplug your bedroom: your bedroom is for two things and two things only. One of them is sleep.
7. Prepare your body for sleep: learn to meditate and/or do simple, restful yoga poses. Goodnight!

RULE 20

PLAN ONE SPLURGE
MEAL A WEEK

"I like the idea of being empowered to make choices, and that includes enjoying it when I make a bad choice AND enjoying it even more when I make a good choice and pass on another bad choice."

—San Antonio *TBL* fan

"I'm a big believer in having a splurge (cheat) meal weekly. Having a splurge meal keeps me on track throughout the week and has helped me to establish my eating program as a lifestyle change instead of a "diet" (quick fix) and is helping eliminate the binge mentality which has plagued me for years. It really works well for me as I have lost 21 pounds so far and curbed my mindless eating and cravings."

—Los Angeles *TBL* fan

"The point is to schedule a "cheat day" or meal—but it's obviously within reason. You don't go out and splurge and blow everything you've achieved in a week. The purpose is, if you want white pasta but you don't normally eat it—then you could have that. You are still totally supposed to stick with proper portion sizes (i.e., not three Big Macs!). Or have that piece of dessert (again, portion!). Some people do better with it, others don't."

—Houston *TBL* fan

I got so much flack when I first started advocating this! People thought I was encouraging a bad pattern—one too similar to your old, binge-fest ways.

And believe me, there are so many ideas about what constitutes a cheat or splurge meal that I had to give a few real-world examples. What is amazing to me is that most weight "losers" understand this. It's really not that complicated if you have been following the Skinny Rules.

The whole idea can be summed up in one word: plan.

Unlike episodic bingeing, splurge meals *are an ingredient in your diet*. When you plan something, *you* are in control. And when you are in control of your splurge, you don't later think that you've failed. And that puts an end to the old binge-shame-diet-binge cycle.

Here are some splurge meal rules:

- You don't get a splurge meal until you've completed the first two weeks of the rules.
- It's *one meal*—breakfast, lunch, or dinner—a week. Not a whole day of splurges!
- Write down the calorie count before you eat.
- You still don't get any liquid calories except red wine. I want you to get used to eating without a sweet drink at hand.

- Decide whether you want to eat rich or eat big. By that I mean, do you want truly forbidden foods (though no fast-food joints!), bigger portions, or some mix? Take note of your answer and write it down on your daily menu. You'll find it tells you a lot about what you really want when you feel deprived.
- Breakfast and lunch are the best times for splurge meals. If you must splurge for dinner, make sure it's before seven (i.e., make a reservation for six o'clock if you're splurging on the town).
- Drink a large glass of water before the meal. At a restaurant order only water and tell them to hold the bread.
- If you are going out to eat, take a look at the restaurant's menu online so you can, you guessed it, make some plans for your meal before you get there.
- You don't get to blow your splurge meal by going to a fast-food place. Eat real food. Barbecue at home. Experiment with a new recipe. Remember, you are changing your life, so start changing your lifestyle. . . .
- Don't splurge by yourself.

PART II

THE SKINNY WAY

All right, you've read the rules—the basic, always-reliable fall-back principles for weight loss.

That is, you'll know what to do when you find yourself in this pickle: Janie's serving tacos and rice for dinner tonight, but it's not your splurge night. You'll remind yourself that *Janie's casa no esta bueno!* Rule 4!

And when you're about to try to convince yourself that because you're in a hurry you should just eat breakfast when you get to work . . . you'll remember Rule 14. And you'll not only eat something nutritious before you leave, you'll also set the alarm a little earlier for tomorrow.

In short, when in doubt, you will do what the rules say. At first, living this way may feel forced, but I promise you that in just a few weeks, the Skinny Rules will have become habit and won't even take conscious thought; they'll have become second nature. I promise. My rules have never let my contestants and clients down, and they'll never let *you* down.

In most diet books this is the part where the author tells you something like: "But don't worry! If you like to eat, it's not the end of the world! I've got a lot of diversity in this diet. You don't have to eat the same thing every day. Why, look at his recipe for lime Jell-O omega-3 parfait!"

But here's the brutal truth: losing weight—and keeping it off—*is* monotonous. Why? Because—particularly at first—you've got to build some *unyielding internal beliefs about how to eat* (habits—what'd I tell you people?!), and you're not going to do that if you get distracted with, well, how to make a lime Jell-O omega-3 parfait. Later, maybe, when you're lighter, tougher-minded, and more confident. For now, you've got to eat like I do.

The point, remember, is to change your life, which starts by changing your lifestyle.

The Skinny Way is organized into five easy pieces: a brief chapter on what you need to do to prepare yourself for success and get organized for the next four weeks, and then four weeks of menu plans. Read "Set Yourself Up for Success" first. In includes lists of things you need to stock up on, food I want you to place at eye level in your fridge from the get-go, and so on. Don't skip this chapter.

The four weekly menu plans will get you through your first, most critical period. You may consider these to be awfully austere. In the first two weeks, they are. But, as I have been harping, I do have a heart. Use a step-down strategy when you need to. And watch how the menus change. They will very slowly ease up and allow you more (in both quantity and diversity) as you progress. Take heart! These four weeks comprise Phase 1 of the rest of your skinny life. My bet is that you will lose so much weight and feel so good that you'll continue following the rules (because, remember, they will be second nature), and you'll need much less daily guidance to do so.

A few notes about the menus:

First, for each meal, the options follow a consistent pattern: there's always a protein (sometimes a non-animal protein—Rule 12!), always a veggie, often a fruit, and, except for dinner, a carbohydrate (because, remember, we're trying to get you to bed a tad hungry—Rule 18). From these menus you will get all the basics that I've outlined in the rules—enough protein and fiber, tons of beneficial nutrients, and a modest amount of energy-boosting, healthy *complex* carbohydrates.

Second, you don't have to eat precisely according to these menus—you can mix and match menus within a given week, and feel free to substitute a menu or recipe from the week before if you loved it and want to eat it again. But don't jump ahead by adding choices from week 3 or week 4 in the first two weeks.

Third, you'll see that I've made separate menu recommendations for women and men. When we're talking about yogurt or berries or hummus or nuts, the amounts are clear in the menus. But when I've referred you to a recipe, you'll have to make your own calculations for what constitutes a serving for you. And you'll base that on gender. Guys need to keep their daily calories around 2,000. Women have to aim for 1,200. This isn't me being sexist. This is a Rule of Nature, folks. Men need more calories. Unfair? Perhaps. But life is unfair. Let's move on.

Fourth, unless specified otherwise, you can eat all the veggies you want, provided they are made according to the rules—roasted, broiled, steamed, stir-fried (so long as you prepare them yourself and use spray oil), or raw. Harpersize them! To repeat: deep-fried, tempura-style, or butter-slathered vegetables (*anything* slathered in butter), would be a big NO.

Finally, remember that even if it feels like I'm giving a lot of directions now, all this *will* soon become second nature. You won't

LIFE IS UNFAIR: WHY IT'S HARDER FOR WOMEN TO LOSE WEIGHT THAN MEN

My plan allows men about 1,500 calories a day. Women get 300 fewer to indulge in. Unfair, you say? No, it's just biology—women need fewer calories.

It turns out that even with fewer calories, women have a harder time losing weight. This doesn't mean that you can't or that you won't. But there are a few things stacked against you that you should be aware of. One of the nutritionists on *The Biggest Loser,* Cheryl Forberg, has a great rap on this topic, and because she happens to fall into the gender that gets the short end of the stick on this topic, I'll let her tell you herself:

Women tend to be more prone to "emotional eating": In 2009, the Brookhaven National Laboratory conducted a brain imaging study to look at how we control our brain responses to our favorite foods. Men were better able to control their responses. This may help explain why women typically have a harder time dropping the pounds.

Men may be more competitive than women: Some research has shown that when money was awarded for every pound lost, men did better. It is interesting to note the percentage of male versus female winners of *The Biggest Loser* (70% of the winners have been male).

Men have more muscle mass: Men tend to have more muscle than women, and we all know that muscle burns more calories than fat. Having a higher muscle composition leads to a higher metabolism. Several studies have shown that a man's metabolism is anywhere from 3 to 10 percent higher than that of a woman of the same weight and age.

Female hormones play a role: Female hormones, such as estrogen, skew your metabolism to deposit fat.

need me telling you to go to the supermarket after Sunday lunch, when you won't be hungry. You won't need me telling you what to place at eye-level in the fridge. And you won't need my constant hectoring about "do this" or "do that."

But for now, do yourself a favor: *Do this! And do that!*

SET YOURSELF UP
FOR SUCCESS

As you'll see as you browse the menus to follow (and as you've figured out if you were paying attention to the rules!), there are four fundamental food groups in my program: protein, vegetables, fruit, and grains. Before you launch into all the great eating to come, it's good to have some general guidelines and information about those four food groups above and beyond the quick overview I gave you in each of the corresponding rules.

Also, I've outlined some things to do *each week* to set yourself up for success. Putting a little time into planning what's going to be on your menu (and therefore in your fridge) will go a very long way toward ensuring you eat what you say you're going to eat.

BECOME A PROTEIN PRO

As you learned in Rule 3, eating more protein is key to your weight loss. You'd think it would be an easy rule to follow—I'm actually telling you to eat *more* of something!

But even if *in theory* it seems easy, you've still got to plan; you've got to invest a little time and energy to succeed with this simple rule.

To prep yourself in the protein department, you need to do the following *every Sunday night* (Saturday works too, of course):

- Hard-boil at least a dozen eggs and put them in a bowl at eye level in your refrigerator. That's where you'll find my eggs— I want them right there when I get a bad craving, so I can peel them quickly and snack on the whites (and, occasionally, the yolks).
- Put your natural nut butters (peanut or almond only) behind something larger in the fridge, so you don't immediately see them when you open the door. It's not that you can't eat these for four weeks, but I'd rather you reach for some other options first. Any time you do dip into nut butters, put the jar back behind something bigger so, again, you'll be less tempted to make it your first choice.
- Put a half dozen 6- to 8-ounce fish fillets, separately wrapped, in the freezer.
- Make one pound of turkey meatballs (see page 168 for a simple recipe) and refrigerate. You'll be eating these a lot.
- Roast four chicken breasts without the skin (see page 167); cut two of them into cubes and refrigerate. These are going to be great on salads.
- Line up seven small (6-ounce) containers of low- or no-fat plain Greek yogurt.
- Make a bowl of hummus (page 170).

Because the following items will keep in your pantry, shop for them once before you get started and buy enough to last the month:

- Cans of water-packed tuna, preferably with easy-lift tops or in sealed bags. (Tins that require a can opener can be sharp and dangerous! Fingers = good. Blood = bad.)
- Canned beans—white, black, garbanzo, and kidney beans (get low-sodium if you're able).
- Bags of dry lentils. Some stores now also sell presteamed and vacuum-packed lentils in the refrigerated produce section (often near the lettuces). These will keep for weeks in your fridge and save you the trouble of cooking (just heat them up if you want warm lentils instead of a cold salad).

> Buy some fresh herbs as well: parsley, basil, and mint add a whole lot of flavor when fresh. But don't chop these herbs ahead of time—make them the last-minute addition so they release their flavor when and where you want it.

VEGGIES AND YOU

My bet is that you have not been eating a lot of vegetables, and if you have, they've been fried, overcooked, salty as hell, and generally disgusting. We're going to change that. Now.

I went over the basics of *why* you need to eat more vegetables in Rule 17, but here let's focus specifically on buying and preparing those vegetables. Let's call these the Veggie Rules.

- Don't stint on quality. It's worth it to spend a little extra on good-quality spinach, be it fresh or frozen. It will taste better.

- When in doubt, buy organic, or, as I like to say, "Be selectively organic." See page 39 for the list of foods I think are worth buying in organic form.
- Be adventurous. Try new veggies. You'll be surprised at what's out there. When you eat them, you'll be happy. Like me. Look at the list below of the veggies I grant you permission to pig out on . . . and the ones you should indulge in a bit more sparingly.
- Store most vegetables in their own refrigerator compartment. Exceptions to the rule—which you should not refrigerate— include tomatoes, peppers, sweet potatoes and squash, and onions. These veggies look nice in a big bowl, and they'll taste better when they are not cold.

AS MUCH AS YOU WANT, ANYTIME VEGGIES

artichoke	fennel
arugula	garden cress
asparagus	green beans
bell peppers	jicama
bok choy	kale
broccoli	kohlrabi
broccoflower	komatsuna (Japanese mustard spinach)
Broccolini	leeks
broccoli rabe	lettuces
broccoli romanesco	mizuna
wild broccoli	mushrooms
Brussels sprouts	mustard greens
cabbage	onions
cauliflower	radishes
chard	spinach
Chinese cabbage	tomatoes
collard greens	yellow summer squash

cucumber   watercress

daikon   zucchini

eggplant

NO MORE THAN HALF A CUP, AND ALWAYS BEFORE 2 P.M.:

beets   rutabaga

carrots   sweet potatoes (and yams)

parsnips   turnips

pumpkin   winter squash (butternut, acorn, Hubbard)

On the vegetable front, here are the things to do every weekend to prepare for easy veggie access all week long:

- Put a plate of Persian cucumbers in the fridge at eye level. How hard was that?
- Make seven large bags of your favorite mixed greens and salad veggies, seal each, and put in the fridge. See where I'm going with this? You'll have no excuses—the salad is ready but for the dressing!

The weekend is also a good time to cook some veggies in advance or try a new technique:

- Experiment with roasting veggies. I've given some guidelines in the recipe section (see pages 176–80). You'll find this method easy, tasty, and quick to clean up. Vegetables roasted over the weekend will stay delicious all week, whether you eat them cold or reheat them. At a minimum, cube three or four small sweet potatoes, put in air-tight bags, and refrigerate so that they'll be ready to roast later in the week.
- Experiment with pan-roasting your vegetables on the stove. A favorite: scorched green beans. Simply trim the tops off the

beans, snap in half, lay in a single layer in a hot, heavy-bottomed fry pan, and let them go for about 8 minutes, tossing occasionally. They'll be slightly blackened and ready for a dose of dressing.

- Try steaming some veggies—it's is a great way to get them ready for a light dressing, but be careful not to steam them so much that they become soggy. When in doubt, take them off the heat!

THE POWER OF PREPARATION

The other night I got home late from work. I was hungry and tired—two danger zones for binge eating, right? My secret saving grace? Preparation. I already had a huge bag of chopped salad ingredients in the refrigerator, so I just dropped the greens in a bowl, dressed them with Galeo's dressing, my favorite, and topped them with the cubed chicken I'd cooked the weekend before. Then I added a lot of cut-up veggies from the extensive list above—some cucumbers, bell peppers, tomatoes, and red onion. Total prep time: just a couple of minutes, which is about all the bandwidth I have left at the end of a long day!

If you chop and bag veggies and a protein ahead of time, you'll be setting yourself up for success big-time. And don't be shy about experimenting with what might seem oddball vegetables in a meal like this. Treat finding new vegetable combinations you like as an adventure!

FRUITS: GO FOR FRESH!

You'll note that except for berries and apples, there's not a lot of fruit on the menu during the first few weeks of the diet. That's because as high as most fruits are in fiber (and berries and apples are especially fibrous), they can be awfully sweet. And a high priority is to break that sweet habit.

But I have a heart! Go ahead and enjoy your fruit but stay away from fruit juices. Remember, we don't want to drink our calories; even no-sugar-added fruit juices don't give you the fiber that you'll get from the actual fruit.

I also want you to stay away from dried fruits: raisins, dried cranberries, cherries, apricots, mangoes . . . you name it: These are basically little sugar bombs! Remember that while a single grape and a single raisin have the same number of calories (3.5), a cup of grapes has 60 calories while a cup of raisins has 400. Solve the dilemma by avoiding them altogether. Eat only fresh fruit!

MY FAVORITE FRUITS

Blueberries

If you were paying attention earlier, you know I want you to eat some berries every day (Rule 6). The blues are so wonderful! One cup contains 3.6 grams of fiber. I always have one or two packages on hand, at least one at eye level in the fridge. Organic: yes.

Apples

Also part of Rule 6 is to eat apples every day. But since apples are a great source of fiber, eating one a day works toward your Rule 5 daily goal as well. One cup of apple slices—one medium apple—contains 3 grams of fiber. Leave a bowl of apples on your counter all the time so that you're encouraged to choose one instead of heading for the refrigerator. One apple is one serving. Fujis are a great choice. Or try some of the newly revived and delicious heirloom apples that have begun appearing at farmer's markets and upscale food stores, such as

Gravenstein and Arkansas Black. Organic: optional (I think organic is worth it here, but I won't insist.)

Strawberries

One cup of whole strawberries has 2.9 grams of fiber. Don't reach for the sugar bowl to sweeten them! Instead, try some low-cal ways to tart them up: a little balsamic vinegar, some ground pepper, a squeeze of lemon juice. Organic: yes.

Avocados

One medium avocado has a whopping 13.2 grams of fiber, or 54 percent of the amount I want you to get a day. But don't eat the whole thing to get that fiber. One-quarter of an avocado per day is your limit—that's still a good step toward your fiber goal. Pump up the flavor with lemon juice. On a splurge day, fill the seed pit cavity with balsamic! Organic: optional.

Bananas

One medium banana contains 3.1 grams of fiber, or 12 percent of my recommended allowance. One small or half a large is your daily limit. Organic: optional.

THE NEW GRAINS

Grains—be they in the form of cereal, pasta, bread, or rice—have not exactly been your friend. At least not your waistline's friend. You know why—we covered that in Rule 4, and that's why you will be giving up all refined grains. Right? It's a big change—but now you get to eat new kinds of grains that fit the rules quite well.

Here is your last set of stocking-up and weekend prep marching orders; then on with the menus.

- Buy microwavable packets of brown rice. You heard me out on Rule 4 about the *relative* virtues of brown rice (better than white rice but still not great), so you know that I don't think it's a great daily go-to choice. If you're going to eat it, at least make sure you're not eating too much. Look for individual-serving microwavable packets—½ cup each, 120 calories, no fat, and 2 grams of fiber. And it tastes great. Get it and make your life easy.
- Stock up on whole-wheat pasta. You know the basics of portion control on this already. Two ounces dry—a dime-size portion if you're cooking spaghetti. And though many people don't think of it, you can make pasta ahead by simply boiling it for one minute less than the package calls for (because you will make up that last minute when you reheat it later), drain and let cool, and put each portion in a sealable bag.

PASTA SERVING SIZES

PASTA SHAPE	UNCOOKED	COOKED
Elbows	½ cup	1 cup
Penne	¾ cup	1 cup
Ribbed lasagna	2½ pieces	2½ pieces
Spaghetti	2 ounces	1¼ cups
Egg noodles	1¼ cups	1¼ cups

- Buy a box or two of farro. Remember, farro is a whole grain that has been used in Italy for centuries. You can cook and use it like rice. Be sure to get the parboiled version; all Italian specialty stores carry it. There are also several online sites (see Resources). It's a bit pricey, but worth every dime because it is so satisfying. Cook it and bag it in ½-cup, 120-calorie servings.
- Buy barley. I know it sounds a little granola-y, but use this great grain! It is inexpensive and fabulously tasty. Get the parboiled version or budget some extra time for prep—just follow the package directions and store it in a sealable bag. Portion: ½ cup cooked. No more.
- Keep quinoa in your pantry. Quinoa is technically a seed, and in recent years has been a hot number with some of the world's leading chefs because of its nutty flavor. It's easy to prepare—simply wash and rinse thoroughly, then boil in water (use amount listed on the package) for about twenty minutes and rinse again. A portion is ½ cup. Don't make too much at one time as it tends to get mushy after a day or so.

Some other grain-preparation tips:

- Dice a variety of vegetables into approximately quarter-inch pieces and mix them into the grains when reheating. You'll feel like you're getting a lot more volume-wise, and you'll be getting a whole lot more nutrition-wise as well.
- Stock up on all kinds of broths—canned low-salt chicken is ideal. Warm up some broth, add a few of those diced veggies and a serving of the grain of your choice, and voilà! Soup. Remember, soup is one of those foods that fills you up without a lot of calories. There are even low-salt veggie bouillon cubes.

BUT WHAT ABOUT THE REST OF THE FAMILY?

One of the more lively conversations in the weight-loss world concerns the family—those members of your household unit who may not need to lose weight. How should we accommodate them? I have one answer: make them a Skinny Rules family! There is nothing in the rules that would be unhealthy for someone of ideal weight. Yes, they can eat more almond butter or beans or steak or bananas or pasta than you, but the principles remain the same. Easy. Right? Well, except for all those special-request items the kids are constantly nagging you about. What's the answer there? I'm afraid that, where food, shopping, health, and kids intersect, you'll find me even more of a hard-ass than usual. In essence: kids don't get a say in what you buy! You are the parent; if you don't buy bad food, they won't eat bad food. I know this flies in the face of today's "never say never to a kid" wisdom, but how's that been working? Childhood obesity rates are higher than ever. So say no. That means: no ice cream in the freezer. (Take them out for some as a treat, but keep it out of the house. You'll scarf it. Trust me. You'll scarf it.) No sugary cereals, crackers, chips, and the like in the pantry. My experience tells me: if something fattening is there, someone will eat it. And that someone will get fat.

THE MENUS

WEEK 1 MENUS

WHAT TO DRINK

As discussed in Rule 1, I want you to stay hydrated. So much so that I feel the need to list water as an item on each menu so that you'll have no excuse for forgetting to just drink the H_2O. That said, in each of these menu options, I include "H_2Ox2" because most glasses are 8-ounce affairs, and you need to get 16 ounces, not 8!

And a note about coffee

I haven't listed coffee or tea as an additional drink option for breakfast, but go ahead and add that to the menu plan if you want! But don't skip the water.

Week 1 Breakfast Options for Women

H₂Ox2
3+1 Omelet (page 162) filled with vegetables
1 slice whole-wheat or whole-grain toast (Ezekiel bread is the best!)
1 cup strawberries

H₂Ox2
1 cup nonfat Greek yogurt with ½ cup berries
1 slice whole-wheat or whole-grain toast

H₂Ox2
½ cup oatmeal
1 sliced apple and 1 cup nonfat Greek yogurt

H₂Ox2
1 slice whole-wheat or whole-grain toast with 1 tablespoon peanut
    or almond butter topped with ½ banana, sliced
1 sliced apple

H₂Ox2
3+1 Omelet (page 162) with 1 teaspoon parmesan cheese sprinkled
    on top
Roasted broccoli and garlic
½ cup berries

H₂Ox2
1 Skinny Shake (page 187)
1 sliced apple
1 cup nonfat Greek yogurt with ½ cup berries and 1 tablespoon pis-
    tachios or almonds

H_2Ox2
½ cup oatmeal
1 cup nonfat Greek yogurt with berries

Week 1 Breakfast Options for Men

H_2Ox2
5+1 Omelet (page 162) filled with vegetables
1 slice whole-wheat or whole-grain toast
1 cup strawberries

H_2Ox2
½ cup nonfat Greek yogurt with ½ cup berries
1 slice whole-wheat or whole-grain toast with a smashed banana
    spread on top

H_2Ox2
½ cup oatmeal with berries
1 sliced apple and 1 tablespoon almond butter

H_2Ox2
1 slice whole-wheat or whole-grain toast with 1 tablespoon peanut
    or almond butter
1 cup nonfat Greek yogurt with ½ cup berries

H_2Ox2
5+1 Omelet (page 162) with 1 teaspoon parmesan cheese sprinkled
    on top
Roasted broccoli and garlic
½ cup berries

> I've mentioned before that when I reach for bread, I reach for the Ezekiel
> brand. It comes in many varieties—all except cinnamon raisin are
> Rules-friendly—and they also now make muffins. In any of my recom-
> mended menus, feel free to use one slice of Ezekiel bread or muffin
> (a half muffin for women, a whole muffin for men) when you see "one
> slice whole-wheat or whole-grain toast."

H_2Ox2
1 Skinny Shake (page 187)
1 sliced apple

H_2Ox2
5+1 Omelet (page 162) with sautéed mushrooms
½ cup oatmeal

Week 1 Midmorning Power Boosts for Women

H_2Ox2
Sliced cucumbers and 1 ounce My Signature No-Oil Hummus (page
    170) or ½ cup nonfat Greek yogurt with lemon and cayenne

H_2Ox2
1 cup blueberries or strawberries
½ cup nonfat ricotta cheese

H_2Ox2
1 sliced apple and 1 ounce hard cheese

H_2Ox2

1 sliced apple and 1 tablespoon peanut butter

H_2Ox2

1 sliced apple and 1 hard-boiled egg

H_2Ox2

1 Skinny Shake (page 187)

H_2Ox2

½ cup nonfat Greek yogurt with ½ cup berries and 1 teaspoon pistachios

---

WHY PERSIAN CUCUMBERS ARE WORTH FINDING

You sure can tell that they're my favorite, right? Why is that? First
reason: they have a distinct, mouth-pleasing taste and crunch. Second:
they are small, and very convenient to cut into slices for dipping or
cubes for salads. They have almost no calories. They are loaded with
fiber. And they are cuter than other varieties.

Week 1 Midmorning Power Boosts for Men

H_2Ox2

Sliced cucumbers and 2 tablespoons My Signature No-Oil Hummus
(page 170) or ½ cup nonfat Greek yogurt with lemon and cayenne

H_2Ox2

1 sliced apple and 1 ounce hard cheese

H_2Ox2
½ cup nonfat Greek yogurt with berries and 1 teaspoon almonds,
pistachios, or walnuts

H_2Ox2
1 sliced apple and 1 tablespoon peanut butter

H_2Ox2
3 hard-boiled egg whites and 1 apple

H_2Ox2
As many raw veggies as you want with a dip of ½ cup nonfat Greek
yogurt and chopped fresh herbs

H_2Ox2
½ apple, ½ banana, and ½ cup blueberries
10 almonds

Week 1 Lunch Options for Women

H_2Ox2
Bob's Cobb (page 173)

H_2Ox2
My Signature Stir-Fry—lunch version—(page 174) with chicken or shrimp
Chopped tomatoes and cucumbers with lemon juice

H_2Ox2
Turkey meatball "sandwich" with tomatoes on lettuce "bun" (see
page 168; use 3 or 4 small meatballs, or 4 ounces turkey)
Roasted vegetable salad

H_2Ox2
Tuna Garbanzo Niçoise Salad (page 223), made with 4 ounces tuna

H_2Ox2
Roasted vegetable salad
Apple, cheese (1 ounce), and cucumber platter

H_2Ox2
1 portion Hearty Tomato-Basil Soup (page 232)
4 ounces chicken or fish, roasted, grilled, or baked

H_2Ox2
Italian Turkey Burger (page 250) on lettuce "buns" with tomato
1 cup berries

Week 1 Lunch Options for Men

H_2Ox2
Italian Turkey Burger (page 250) on lettuce "buns," with nonfat
    Greek yogurt and fresh herbs as your condiment
Large salad of cucumbers, tomatoes, sliced fennel, and lemon juice

H_2Ox2
Jumbo Tuna Garbanzo Niçoise Salad (page 223), made with
    6 ounces tuna

H_2Ox2
Turkey meatball "sandwich" (using 5 ounces turkey or about 5 small
    meatballs) with tomato and onion on lettuce "bun" (see page
    168)
Scorched green beans (see page 104) with mustard dressing

H_2Ox2

Roasted veggie salad with 4 ounces cubed chicken

My Signature No-Oil Hummus (page 170) and cucumber slices

H_2Ox2

Black beans and 4 ounces chicken, tossed with 1 teaspoon olive oil
and lemon juice on lettuce "bun"

Tomato, red onion, cucumber, and feta (½ ounce, crumbled) with
lemon or lime juice and cracked pepper

H_2Ox2

Simple fish and greens soup (see core Roasted Fish recipe,
page 164)

Tomato, cucumber, and onion salad with lemon juice and black
pepper

H_2Ox2

Bob's Cobb (page 173)

Week 1 Midafternoon Power Boosts for Women

H_2Ox2

1 apple and 1 ounce cheese

H_2Ox2

Cucumber slices and 2 tablespoons My Signature No-Oil Hummus
(page 170)

H_2Ox2

Berries and ½ cup nonfat Greek yogurt

H_2Ox2
2 Turkey Meatballs (page 168) with tomatoes and lettuce "bun"

H_2Ox2
1 sliced apple sprinkled with cinnamon and 1 cup nonfat Greek yogurt

H_2Ox2
1 small Mean, Green Drink (½ recipe, page 188)

H_2Ox2
Up to 2 cups mixed berries and apple slices

Week 1 Midafternoon Power Boosts for Men

H_2Ox2
1 sliced apple and 2 ounces cheese

H_2Ox2
Cucumber slices and 2 tablespoons My Signature No-Oil Hummus
   (page 170)

H_2Ox2
½ cup nonfat Greek yogurt with ½ cup berries

H_2Ox2
3 Turkey Meatballs (page 168) with tomatoes

H_2Ox2
4 hard-boiled egg whites
Raw veggies

H_2Ox2
1 Mean, Green Drink (page 188)

H_2Ox2
½ cup herbed nonfat Greek yogurt with tomatoes, cucumbers, and
  black pepper

Week 1 Dinner Options for Women

H_2Ox2
6 ounces fish in tomato puree (pureed Roasted Tomatoes, page 177)
Roasted Cauliflower (page 180) and green beans with lemon juice
  and 1 teaspoon olive oil

H_2Ox2
4 Turkey Meatballs (page 168) and sautéed spinach in chicken broth
Mixed tomato and greens salad

H_2Ox2
4 to 6 ounces Pesto-Roasted Chicken Breast (see page 257)
Green beans with lemon juice and 1 teaspoon olive oil

H_2Ox2
6 ounces (white fish) or 4 ounces (salmon) Fish Ka-Bobs with peppers, tomatoes, and squash (page 259)
Roasted Cauliflower (page 180) or Braised Rapini (page 181)

H_2Ox2
My Signature Stir-Fry—dinner version (page 174)
Salad of cucumber, tomato, and 1 ounce feta, crumbled

H_2Ox2
3+1 Veggie Frittata (page 163)
Roasted Tomatoes, blended for a soup (page 177)

H_2Ox2
4 ounces steak, grilled
Asparagus and tomatoes with lemon juice and 1 teaspoon olive oil

Week 1 Dinner Options for Men

H_2Ox2
8 ounces fish in tomato broth (see page 189)
Roasted Cauliflower (page 180) with green beans and lemon juice–
    olive oil dressing

H_2Ox2
6 Turkey Meatballs (page 168) and spinach sautéed in chicken
    broth
Tomato and mixed greens salad

H_2Ox2
8 ounces Pesto-Roasted Chicken Breast (page 257)
Roasted green beans with 1 teaspoon chopped pistachios

H_2Ox2
8 ounces (white) or 6 ounces (salmon) Fish Ka-Bobs (page 259)
    with peppers, tomatoes, and squash
Roasted Cauliflower (page 180) with Chili Dressing (page 183) or
    Braised Rapini (page 181)

H_2Ox2
My Signature Stir-Fry—dinner version (page 174)
Salad of cucumber, tomato, and 1 ounce feta, crumbled

H_2Ox2
6 ounces steak, grilled
Asparagus and tomatoes with lemon juice and herb vinaigrette

H_2Ox2
5+1 Veggie Frittata (page 163)
Tomatoes, arugula, and cucumbers with chili flakes and a squeeze of
   orange juice

WEEK 2 MENUS

Week 2 Breakfast Options for Women

H_2Ox2
3+1 Omelet (page 162)
2 to 3 ounces Roasted Yam Hashbrowns (page 176)
1 cup berries

H_2Ox2
½ cup oatmeal with berries
1 sliced apple with ½ cup nonfat Greek yogurt

H_2Ox2
3+1 Omelet (page 162) with spinach and 1 tablespoon parmesan
    sprinkled on top or cooked in
1 slice toast with ½ banana smashed and spread on top

H_2Ox2
1 slice toast with 1 tablespoon almond butter and ½ banana, sliced
½ cup blueberries

H_2Ox2
Skinny Shake (page 187)
1 slice toast

H_2Ox2
½ cup oatmeal with ½ cup berries
½ cup nonfat Greek yogurt with ½ banana

H_2Ox2
1 ounce hard cheese
1 sliced apple
1 slice toast

Week 2 Breakfast Options for Men

H_2Ox2
5+1 Omelet (page 162)
½ cup Roasted Yam Hashbrowns (page 176) OR 1 slice bread
1 cup blueberries

H_2Ox2
4 hard-boiled egg whites
1 slice toast
1 small apple and 1 cup nonfat Greek yogurt

H_2Ox2
½ cup oatmeal with berries
3+1 Omelet (page 162)

H_2Ox2
5+1 Omelet (page 162) with spinach
1 slice toast
1 cup strawberries

H_2Ox2
1 slice toast with 1 tablespoon almond butter and ½ banana, sliced
1 sliced apple

H_2Ox2
Skinny Shake (page 187)
1 slice toast

H_2Ox2
3+1 Veggie Frittata (page 163) with 1 ounce grated cheese on top
1 slice toast
½ cup berries

Week 2 Midmorning Power Boosts for Women

H_2Ox2
2 tablespoons My Signature No-Oil Hummus (page 170) and cucumber slices

H_2Ox2
Raw veggies and ½ cup herbed and peppered nonfat Greek yogurt

H_2Ox2
1 sliced apple and 1 ounce cheddar cheese

H_2Ox2
1 cup berries, ½ cup nonfat Greek yogurt, and 1 tablespoon pistachios

H_2Ox2
1 sliced apple and 1 tablespoon almond butter

H_2Ox2
Skinny Shake (page 187)

H_2Ox2
1 cup berries and ½ cup nonfat Greek yogurt sprinkled with cinnamon

Week 2 Midmorning Power Boosts for Men

H_2Ox2
3 tablespoons My Signature No-Oil Hummus (page 170) and cucumber slices

H_2Ox2
Raw veggies and ½ cup herbed and peppered nonfat Greek yogurt

H_2Ox2
1 sliced apple and 1 ounce cheddar cheese

H_2Ox2
1 sliced apple and 1 tablespoon almond butter

H_2Ox2
1 cup berries, ½ cup nonfat Greek yogurt, and 1 tablespoon pistachios

H_2Ox2
5 hard-boiled egg whites
Cucumber and tomato slices with lemon and black pepper

H_2Ox2
Skinny Shake (page 187)

Week 2 Lunch Options for Women

H_2Ox2

Roasted asparagus and red bell pepper and 1 chopped hard-boiled
   egg on top

2 tablespoons My Signature No-Oil Hummus (page 170) and cucumber strips

H_2Ox2

Roasted tomato halves stuffed with "Makes Me Happy" Tuna Salad
   (page 166)

Apple and roasted Jerusalem artichoke salad with Galeo's dressing
   or one of my Core dressings (see pages 182–86)

H_2Ox2

Chicken broth with tomatoes, garbanzos, and veggies

H_2Ox2

3+1 onion, pepper, and egg frittata (hot or cold, see
   page 163)

My Signature No-Oil Hummus (page 170) and pepper strips

H_2Ox2

4 Turkey Meatballs (page 168) in tomato or chicken broth (see page
   189), topped with parmesan

Large green salad with peppers and 1 tablespoon garbanzo
   beans

H_2Ox2

My Signature Stir-Fry—lunch version (page 174)

H_2Ox2

4 ounces cubed chicken, mixed with 1 teaspoon pistachios and
your choice of dressing (pages 182–186)

As many raw veggies as you want

Week 2 Lunch Options for Men

H_2Ox2

Chicken soup with tomatoes, garbanzos, and veggies with 1 tablespoon parmesan cheese sprinkled on top

1 slice toast

H_2Ox2

5+1 onion, pepper, and egg frittata (hot or cold, see page 163)

My Signature No-Oil Hummus (page 170) and cucumber strips

H_2Ox2

5 Turkey Meatballs (page 168) in tomato or chicken broth (see
page 189), topped with parmesan

Large green salad with peppers and 1 tablespoon garbanzo
beans

H_2Ox2

French Chicken Salad Lettuce Wraps (page 222)

1 cup berries and sliced apple

H_2Ox2

1 portion Hearty Tomato-Basil Soup (page 222)

Tomato and cucumbers mixed with arugula and lemon juice

H_2O x2
1 portion My Signature Stir-Fry—lunch version (page 174)
1 cup blueberries

H_2O x2
The Leanburger (page 169)

Week 2 Midafternoon Power Boosts for Women

H_2O x2
1 cup berries with ½ cup nonfat Greek yogurt

H_2O x2
2 tablespoons My Signature No-Oil Hummus (page 170) with
   lemon, tomato, and cucumbers

H_2O x2
1 sliced apple and 1 ounce hard cheese

H_2O x2
1 sliced apple and 1 tablespoon peanut butter

H_2O x2
Skinny Shake (page 187)

H_2O x2
Raw veggies and ½ cup herbed and peppered nonfat Greek yogurt

H_2O x2
1 cup berries, ½ cup nonfat Greek yogurt, and 1 tablespoon
   pistachios

Week 2 Midafternoon Power Boosts for Men

H₂Ox2
1 apple, 10 almonds, and 1 ounce hard cheese

H₂Ox2
3 tablespoons My Signature No-Oil Hummus (page 170) and cucumber slices

H₂Ox2
Raw veggies and ½ cup herbed and peppered nonfat Greek
yogurt

H₂Ox2
1 sliced apple and 1 tablespoon almond butter

H₂Ox2
Berries, ½ cup nonfat Greek yogurt, and 1 tablespoon pistachios

H₂Ox2
5 hard-boiled egg whites
Cucumber and tomato slices with lemon and black pepper

H₂Ox2
1 sliced apple and 1 tablespoon peanut butter

Week 2 Dinner Options for Women

H₂Ox2
My Signature Stir-Fry—dinner version (page 174) with chicken

H_2Ox2
Fish Ka-Bobs (page 259)
Roasted vegetables and mixed greens (see page 58)

H_2Ox2
My Signature Stir-Fry (174) with shrimp or chicken
Fennel, bell pepper, and onion salad with lemon and black
    pepper

H_2Ox2
Bob's Cobb (page 173)

H_2Ox2
3+1 Veggie Frittata (page 163)
Apple and fennel salad with ground hemp seeds

H_2Ox2
5-ounce Italian Turkey Burger (page 250) with tomatoes, onions,
    and lettuce "buns"
String beans in Mustard Vinaigrette (page 184)

H_2Ox2
4 to 6 ounces Pesto-Roasted Chicken Breast (page 257)
Green beans with lemon juice and 1 teaspoon olive oil

Week 2 Dinner Options for Men

H_2Ox2
My Signature Stir-Fry—dinner verison (page 174) with
    shrimp

H_2Ox2
Fish Ka-Bobs (page 259)
Roasted veggies over mixed greens and 1 tablespoon of one of my
    dressings

H_2Ox2
My Signature Stir-Fry—dinner version (page 174) with tofu
Harpersized fennel, pepper, and onion salad

H_2Ox2
Bob's Cobb (page 173)

H_2Ox2
3+1 Veggie Frittata (page 163)
Apple and fennel salad with lemon juice and 1 teaspoon olive oil

H_2Ox2
6-ounce Italian Turkey Burger (page 250) with ½ ounce cheddar
    and tomato on lettuce "bun"
String beans in Mustard Vinaigrette (page 184)

H_2Ox2
Pesto-Roasted Chicken Breast (page 257)
Spinach and apple salad with lemon juice and olive oil dressing

WEEK 3 MENUS

Can we just pause for a moment? You are now midway through the first—and most crucial—period of rules-based eating.

Congratulations, I know that weight loss—especially in the beginning—is tedious, repetitive, and somewhat dull. I told you that right from the start. The path to obesity is paved with bacon and white bread; the way to skinny is built on apples and Ezekiel! But if you persist, I promise you two things: you'll develop a tough, skinny-eating mind-set for the future, and, of course, you'll lose weight.

Also, from here on you're going to start seeing more variety.

Week 3 Breakfast Options for Women

H_2Ox2
Apple Berry Yogurt Shake (page 212)
1 slice toast

H_2Ox2
B.E.S.T. Breakfast Sandwich (page 191)

H_2Ox2
Berry salad with Balsamic Dressing (page 182)
1 slice toast with 1 tablespoon peanut butter

H_2Ox2
3+1 Omelet (page 162) with ¼ avocado
1 cup strawberries

H_2Ox2
½ cup Roasted Yam Hashbrowns (page 176)
½ cup nonfat Greek yogurt with ½ cup blueberries

H_2Ox2

½ cup Fall Pumpkin Oatmeal (page 204)

½ cup nonfat Greek yogurt or 3 hard-boiled egg whites

H_2Ox2

1 slice toast topped with 1 tablespoon peanut butter and ½ banana, sliced

Week 3 Breakfast Options for Men

H_2Ox2

Apple Berry Yogurt Shake (page 212)

1 slice toast

H_2Ox2

1 sliced apple and nonfat Greek yogurt

5+1 Omelet (page 162)

H_2Ox2

½ cup Fall Pumpkin Oatmeal (page 204)

½ cup nonfat Greek yogurt or 5 hard-boiled egg whites

H_2Ox2

Berry salad with Balsamic Dressing (page 182)

1 slice toast with 1 tablespoon peanut butter

H_2Ox2

5+1 Omelet (page 162) with ¼ avocado

½ cup strawberries

H_2Ox2
B.E.S.T. Breakfast Sandwich (page 191)

H_2Ox2
Skinny Shake (page 187)
1 slice toast

Week 3 Midmorning Power Boosts for Women
– –

H_2Ox2
2 tablespoons My Signature No-Oil Hummus (page 170) with cucumbers, red peppers, and jicama sticks

H_2Ox2
½ small avocado mashed with lemon and cayenne, with red pepper
strips

H_2Ox2
1 cup berries and 1 cup nonfat Greek yogurt

H_2Ox2
1 medium apple, sliced, with 1 tablespoon almond or peanut butter

H_2Ox2
Skinny Shake (page 187)

H_2Ox2
½ cup herbed nonfat Greek yogurt dip
Cucumber and red pepper strips

H_2Ox2
1 sliced apple with 1 tablespoon almond or peanut butter

Week 3 Midmorning Power Boosts for Men

H_2Ox2
Celery sticks and 1 tablespoon peanut butter or 2 tablespoons My
Signature No-Oil Hummus (page 170)

H_2Ox2
½ small avocado mashed with lemon and cayenne, with red pepper
strips

H_2Ox2
Skinny Shake (page 187)

H_2Ox2
5 hard-boiled egg whites
Celery, cucumber, and red pepper strips

H_2Ox2
½ cup nonfat Greek yogurt with ½ cup berries

H_2Ox2
3 tablespoons My Signature No-Oil Hummus (page 170)
red pepper strips

H_2Ox2
1 sliced apple and 1 tablespoon almond butter

Week 3 Lunch Options for Women

H_2Ox2
Bob's Cobb (page 173) with strawberries and ¼ avocado added,
cheese omitted

H_2Ox2
4 ounces chicken cubes, 1 tablespoon walnuts, lemon juice, and pa-
prika or black pepper
Basic green salad

H_2Ox2
Hearty Tomato-Basil Soup (page 232) with chicken cubes and a dab
of nonfat Greek yogurt
Berries and an apple

H_2Ox2
3+1 Veggie Frittata with mushrooms (page 163) with 1 teaspoon
parmesan sprinkled on top
Berries and an apple

H_2Ox2
My Signature Stir-Fry—lunch version (page 174)

H_2Ox2
Curried Chicken and Quinoa Salad (page 228)

H_2Ox2
Savory Lentil Soup (page 233)

Week 3 Lunch Options for Men

H_2Ox2
5+1 spinach and kale frittata (page 163)
1 sliced apple and berries

H_2Ox2
Bob's Cobb (page 173), with strawberries and ¼ avocado added,
    cheese omitted

H_2Ox2
6 ounces cubed chicken with diced tomatoes, red bell pepper,
    lemon, and paprika
Basic green salad

H_2Ox2
Hearty Tomato-Basil Soup (page 232) with chicken cubes
1 sliced apple and berries

H_2Ox2
Curried Chicken and Quinoa Salad (page 228)

H_2Ox2
Savory Lentil Soup (page 233)

H_2Ox2
The Leanburger (page 169)

Week 3 Midafternoon Power Boosts for Women

H_2Ox2
Berry and apple Skinny Shake (page 187)

H_2Ox2
2 tablespoons My Signature No-Oil Hummus (page 170) and cucumbers

H_2Ox2
1 cup berries with balsamic vinegar and mint, dab of nonfat Greek yogurt, and 1 teaspoon crushed pistachios, walnuts, or almonds

H_2Ox2
Nonfat Greek yogurt with berries and 10 nuts

H_2Ox2
½ cup herbed nonfat Greek yogurt dip
½ apple, sliced

H_2Ox2
1 ounce hard cheese
Cucumber and pepper strips

H_2Ox2
½ apple, sliced
1 tablespoon peanut butter

Week 3 Midafternoon Power Boosts for Men

H_2Ox2
Berry and apple Skinny Shake (page 187)

H_2Ox2
2 tablespoons My Signature No-Oil Hummus (page 170) and cu-
    cumbers

H_2Ox2
1 cup berries with balsamic vinegar, mint, and a dab of nonfat
    Greek yogurt

H_2Ox2
1 cup nonfat Greek yogurt with berries and 10 nuts

H_2Ox2
½ cup herbed yogurt dip
1 sliced apple

H_2Ox2
1 ounce hard cheese
Cucumber and pepper strips

H_2Ox2
1 sliced apple
1 tablespoon peanut butter

Week 3 Dinner Options for Women

H_2Ox2
6 ounces Fish Ka-Bobs (page 259)
Braised Broccoli (page 181)
Cucumber, pepper, and tomatoes

H_2Ox2
4 Turkey Meatballs (page 168) with roasted peppers and green
    beans
Spinach and strawberry salad with balsamic and 1 teaspoon
    olive oil

H_2Ox2
Chicken broth with shredded chicken and 1 tablespoon parmesan
    cheese (page 189)
Giant mix of your favorite veggies, stir-fried

H_2Ox2
Roasted Tomatoes (page 177) with shrimp or tofu
Grilled Asparagus (page 179) and hard-boiled egg-white salad

H_2Ox2
4 ounces steak, roasted, with Roasted Tomatoes (page 177)
Basic green salad with lemon and 1 teaspoon olive oil

H_2Ox2
4 ounces Herb-Roasted Chicken Breast (page 167)
Grilled Asparagus (page 179) with lemon and black pepper
Basic green salad

H_2Ox2
4 ounces Beef Ka-Bobs (page 258)
Grilled Asparagus (page 179)
Cucumber, pepper, and tomatoes

Week 3 Dinner Options for Men

H_2Ox2
6 ounces Beef Ka-Bobs (page 258)
Cucumber, pepper, and tomatoes

H_2Ox2
5 Turkey Meatballs (page 168) with roasted peppers and green beans
Spinach and strawberry salad with lemon and 1 teaspoon olive oil

H_2Ox2
Your Own Chicken Broth with shredded chicken added back in, and
    1 tablespoon parmesan (see 189)
Giant veggie stir-fry

H_2Ox2
6 ounces Fish Ka-Bobs (page 259)
Braised Broccoli (page 181)
Cucumber, pepper, and tomatoes

H_2Ox2
Roasted Tomatoes (page 177) with shrimp or tofu
Grilled Asparagus (page 179) and hard-boiled egg-white salad
Basic green salad

H_2Ox2
4 ounces steak, roasted, with Roasted Tomatoes (page 177)
Basic green salad with lemon and 1 teaspoon olive oil

H_2Ox2
4-ounce roasted chicken breast
Roasted or steamed asparagus with lemon and black pepper
Basic green salad

WEEK 4 MENUS

Things may be feeling a little easier now. You're getting used to the rules and perhaps they are becoming a habit. Good. In week 4, you'll see the gradual return of grains to your diet. Small amounts of grain, but remember that you're trying to *lose* weight here. When you're in *maintenance* mode, you can add more.

Week 4 Breakfast Options for Women

H_2Ox2
3+1 Veggie Frittata (page 163) with herbs and nonfat Greek yogurt
½ cup oatmeal with berries

H_2Ox2
½ cup oatmeal
½ cup nonfat Greek yogurt and berries

H_2Ox2
1 slice toast topped with 1 tablespoon almond or peanut butter and
   ½ banana, sliced
½ cup berries

H_2Ox2
1 slice toast
Apple, berries, and 1 ounce cheese

H_2Ox2
Skinny Shake (page 187)
1 slice toast

H_2Ox2

3+1 Omelet (page 162)

½ cup Roasted Yam Hashbrowns (page 176)

½ cup berries

H_2Ox2

½ cup Fall Pumpkin Oatmeal (page 204)

½ cup berries

Week 4 Breakfast Options for Men

H_2Ox2

5+1 Omelet (page 162) with veggies

1 slice toast

1 sliced apple

H_2Ox2

½ cup oatmeal

1 cup nonfat Greek yogurt with berries

H_2Ox2

1 slice toast topped with 1 tablespoon almond or peanut butter and
½ banana, sliced

H_2Ox2

Skinny Shake (page 187)

1 slice toast

H_2Ox2

½ cup Fall Pumpkin Oatmeal (page 204)

1 cup nonfat Greek yogurt with ½ cup berries

H_2Ox2
1 slice toast with 1 tablespoon nut butter
1 cup berries

H_2Ox2
5+1 Omelet (page 162) with veggies
1 slice toast
½ cup berries

Week 4 Midmorning Power Boosts for Women

H_2Ox2
½ cup nonfat Greek yogurt with 1 cup berries

H_2Ox2
Skinny Shake (page 187)

H_2Ox2
1 sliced apple with 1 tablespoon peanut butter

H_2Ox2
2 tablespoons My Signature No-Oil Hummus (page 170) and raw
   veggie slices

H_2Ox2
1 cup berries, balsamic, mint, 1 tablespoon nonfat Greek yogurt,
   and 3 walnut halves, crumbled

H_2Ox2
2 tablespoons My Signature No-Oil Hummus (page 170) and cucumbers

H_2Ox2
Skinny Shake (page 187)

Week 4 Midmorning Power Boosts for Men

H_2Ox2
Skinny Shake (page 187)

H_2Ox2
3 tablespoons My Signature No-Oil Hummus (page 170) and cucumber slices

H_2Ox2
1 cup nonfat Greek yogurt with ½ cup blueberries and 3 walnut halves, crumbled

H_2Ox2
1 cup berries with balsamic vinegar, mint, and a dab of nonfat Greek yogurt

H_2Ox2
1 cup nonfat Greek yogurt with ½ cup berries and 10 nuts

H_2Ox2
½ cup herbed nonfat Greek yogurt dip
1 sliced apple

H_2Ox2
1 ounce hard cheese
Cucumber and pepper strips

Week 4 Lunch Options for Women

H_2Ox2
2 ounces (dry) whole-wheat spaghetti with 4 ounces cubed chicken
    breast tossed with lemon juice, tomatoes, and parsley, sprinkled
    with parmesan cheese

H_2Ox2
Large bowl roasted tomato soup with 4 ounces cubed chicken and
    garbanzo beans on top as croutons
Greens and raw veggie salad

H_2Ox2
Mushroom Barley Soup (page 231)
1 cup berries mixed with diced cucumbers and balsamic dressing

H_2Ox2
Tuna-Farro-Veggie Salad (page 226)

H_2Ox2
Brown rice or Farro Stir-Fry (page 227)

H_2Ox2
Savory Lentil Soup (page 233)
½ cup nonfat Greek yogurt with ½ cup berries

H_2Ox2
2 Ahi Tacos with Mango Salad (page 216)
Bell pepper and cucumber strips

Week 4 Lunch Options for Men

H_2Ox2
2 Ahi Tacos with Mango Salad (page 216)
Bell pepper and cucumber strips

H_2Ox2
2 ounces (dry) whole-wheat spaghetti with 4 ounces cubed chicken
    breast tossed with lemon, garlic, and parsley, sprinkled with par-
    mesan cheese

H_2Ox2
Large bowl roasted tomato soup with 4 ounces cubed chicken and
    garbanzo beans as croutons
Large salad of greens and raw veggies

H_2Ox2
Mushroom Barley (or pasta) Soup (page 231)
Green beans with Galeo's salad dressing

H_2Ox2
Tuna-Farro-Veggie Salad (page 226)

H_2Ox2
Brown rice or Farro Stir-Fry (page 227)
Tomato and cucumber salad

H_2Ox2
2 Eggplant Pizza Muffins (page 224)

Week 4 Midafternoon Power Boosts for Women

H$_2$Ox2
3 hard-boiled egg whites and raw veggies

H$_2$Ox2
1 sliced apple and 1 ounce cheddar or 2 ounces mozzarella

H$_2$Ox2
2 tablespoons My Signature No-Oil Hummus (page 170) with cucumber and pepper slices

H$_2$Ox2
½ cup herbed nonfat Greek yogurt dip with raw veggies

H$_2$Ox2
Celery strips with 1 tablespoon almond butter

H$_2$Ox2
2 Turkey Meatballs (page 168) on lettuce cups
Raw veggies

H$_2$Ox2
2 cups berries
½ cup nonfat Greek yogurt

Week 4 Midafternoon Power Boosts for Men

H$_2$Ox2
5 hard-boiled egg whites and raw veggies

H_2Ox2

1 sliced apple and 1 ounce cheddar or 2 ounces mozzarella

H_2Ox2

2 tablespoons My Signature No-Oil Hummus (page 170) with cucumber and pepper slices

H_2Ox2

½ cup herbed nonfat Greek yogurt dip with raw veggies

H_2Ox2

Celery strips with 1 tablespoon almond butter

H_2Ox2

2 Turkey Meatballs (page 168) on lettuce cups
Raw veggies

H_2Ox2

½ cup nonfat Greek yogurt with berries

Week 4 Dinner Options for Women

H_2Ox2

4-ounce Italian Turkey Burger (page 250) with Roasted Tomatoes
(page 177) as a condiment
Large roasted veggie salad
1 cup chicken broth

H_2Ox2

4 ounces lean steak, roasted, with Pesto (page 185)
Scorched green beans with Mustard Sauce (page 186)

H₂Ox2

Ka-Bobs made with 4 ounces chicken or salmon, or 6 ounces white
   fish (see page 259)

Harpersized mixed greens salad

H₂Ox2

3+1 herb and spinach frittata (page 163) with Roasted Tomatoes
   (page 177)

Pepper, red onion, and arugula salad

H₂Ox2

3 French Chicken Salad Lettuce Wraps (page 222)

½ cup each blueberries and strawberries

H₂Ox2

Bob's Cobb (page 173)

H₂Ox2

Hearty Tomato-Basil Soup (page 232)

Week 4 Dinner Options for Men

H₂Ox2

6-ounce Italian Turkey Burger (page 250) with Roasted Tomatoes
   (page 177)

Cucumber, apple, and fennel strips with lemon juice and black pepper

H₂Ox2

4 ounces lean steak with Pesto (page 185)

Arugula, tomato, and pepper salad

H_2Ox2
Ka-Bobs made with 6 ounces chicken or salmon, or 8 ounces white
 fish (see page 259)
Harpersized mixed greens salad

H_2Ox2
5+1 herb and spinach frittata (page 163) with Roasted Tomatoes
 (page 177)
Pepper, red onion, and arugula salad

H_2Ox2
Bob's Cobb (page 173)
Grilled Asparagus (page 179)

H_2Ox2
Hearty Tomato-Basil Soup (page 232)
Dinner salad with your choice of my dressings

H_2Ox2
Roasted Tomatoes (page 177) with shrimp
Grilled Asparagus (page 179) and hard-boiled egg-white salad
Basic green salad

PART III

THE SKINNY TOOLS

O K, let's refresh: you've read the Skinny Rules and have committed to making them a part of your life. You've read the Skinny Way and are now ready to start your month of rules menus. In this section, I offer you the tools, recipes, and tips that correspond to some of my suggested menus and that will help you use the rules *to get skinny.*

A few things to note before you launch in:

ONE: As you may have figured out in reading the menus, many of my suggestions are variations on the same theme; they build off the same foundation ingredients and techniques. Which means that the recipes to pay attention to at the outset are my "core" recipes. Learn these foundation recipes and you'll have a launching pad for your own easy, tasty repertoire. And you'll always know the recipe follows my rules. I wouldn't put it there if it didn't. Once you've mastered my core recipes (OK, at least read them), check out the recipes organized by meal type (breakfast, lunch, dinner) that follow.

TWO: Recipe yields vary so pay attention! If you're cooking for more than yourself, you may need to double or triple a recipe accordingly. If you're cooking for just little ole you, pay attention to how much each recipe yields. You may be surprised—some will seem "small," but this is just because most of us have a warped sense of the appropriate amount of food to heap on our plates. Some recipes, though, will seem huge—remember, you can Harpersize many vegetables, and when you do that, your plate will be overflowing! But you'll also see how *much* of some foods you can have without any weight gain.

THREE: Read the entire recipe all the way through, and gather all the ingredients before proceeding. If my directions seem overly obvious in places, don't take offense. I'm simply trying to make the process easier and clearer, especially for those of you who've never or rarely cooked.

FOUR: I have tried to insert vegan and vegetarian ingredient options, but in some cases animal fats or proteins are so important that I'd be misleading you if I suggested you could get by without them. No doubt I'll get a million e-mails disagreeing with me on this. I appreciate your input. Please tell me *your* recipe suggestions and I'll give them a try! If I love your recipe, I may post it on my website.

FIVE: Have fun with these recipes! If you're not in the habit of cooking for yourself, approach these recipes with the same mind-set you would when commencing a new workout—you won't get it perfect the first time, but that shouldn't stop you from trying again! I mention this because so many people are actually afraid of cooking, as if it is some magic skill that must be learned in an expensive cooking school. Not so with my recipes! Most can be done in less than one hour, prep time included.

THE FACTS ABOUT FATS

All fats, whether lard, butter, margarine, or olive oil, have the same calorie count: 120 per tablespoon. If we're going to cook with them, we've got to cook smart. We'll use the healthy oils listed below, and we'll use them strategically.

First: use olive or canola oil spray! A few sprays onto a pan before making an omelet adds almost no calories and makes cleanup a breeze.

Second: remember that a little olive oil goes a long way. For dressings, one teaspoon of oil to two teaspoons of lemon juice = a tasty 40-calorie dressing that will be good on any salad you can dream up.

Third: A great way to control (and reduce) the amount of oil you use is to use a spray oil. Since not all oils come in a spray, buy a spray bottle or mister and fill it with oil to make your own.

Last, experiment! Try mixing your favorite citrus juices (lime, grapefruit, orange) with small amounts of oil as a way to flavor soups, veggies, meats, and fish. Play around with fresh herbs as well. My bet is that you'll end up with your own favorite concoctions that make eating the Skinny Way also eating the tasty way!

My Oils and How I Use Them

- For basic pan-searing and browning, I use canola oil; note that it does not add taste.
- For salads and uncooked veggies in general, I use olive oil, the king of healthy oils. Use the expensive extra virgin stuff on salads, and the more affordable versions for everything else.
- For stir-frying, try canola oil (high in omega-6s) or peanut oil.
- If you want to impart a nutty flavor, use toasted sesame oil.
- Use avocado oil on salads and all raw veggie snacks.
- I use walnut and almond oil sparingly on all raw veggies, and for light sautéing.

THE CORE RECIPES

PROTEINS

By now you know how important protein is for your weight loss. If you've forgotten, here is the cheat sheet: protein makes you feel full longer, so you are less likely to slip and eat too much or eat the wrong thing. Protein helps keep blood sugar and insulin in check, making it easier to maintain weight loss and keeping chronic diseases like diabetes and high cholesterol at bay. And protein fuels muscle mass; muscles burn more calories than fat. This is a good thing.

EGGS

5+1 (for men) or 3+1 (for women) Omelet

INGREDIENTS

5 or 3 large eggs, separated
Olive oil or canola oil spray

DIRECTIONS

1. Separate the eggs: Put out two breakfast bowls. Crack each egg on the counter, then let the egg white dribble into one of the bowls as you pass the yolk from one half to the other. Put the yolk in the other bowl.
2. When you crack the last egg, put the entire egg (yolk and white) into the egg white bowl, so there are a lot of egg whites and one yolk. Add a pinch of pepper and any other herb you like and whisk the eggs.
3. Scramble them up: Spray a pan with oil, heat it over medium heat, and pour in the eggs. Here you can decide to make it fast and easy for yourself and simply cook the eggs by continuing to stir them—scrambled eggs—or don't disturb them and let them cook about halfway through. Then, using a spatula, fold what is basically a giant egg patty in half.
4. Cook another few minutes, then slide it onto your plate.

NUTRITION INFORMATION:

5+1 = 146 calories, 25g protein, 0g carbs, 4.4g fat
3+1 = 112 calories, 17.5g protein, 0g carbs, 4.4g fat

Veggie Frittata

INGREDIENTS

Olive oil spray

5/3+1 Omelet mixture (preceding recipe)

As many green leafy veggies and mushrooms as you like

DIRECTIONS

1. Preheat the broiler.
2. Meanwhile, put a large skillet over high heat on the stove. Spray the skillet with olive oil.
3. Place the leafy greens in the skillet and let them wilt. Turn the heat to medium-low.
4. Pour the eggs over the greens and let the mixture cook slowly, lifting up the edges occasionally to check that the frittata is not burning.
5. When the eggs appear almost done, place the pan under the broiler. Check after a minute: the top should just be beginning to brown.
6. Remove from the broiler, set the pan on the stove, and let sit for a few minutes; then slide the frittata onto a plate. Eat immediately.

Or, you could also:

- Let it get cold, wrap in plastic, and refrigerate. Take it to work tomorrow mixed with tomatoes, garbanzo beans, and a little dressing. Delicious!
- Cut the cold frittata in long strips for use on top of salads. Put the strips in a covered container or on a covered plate set at eye level in your refrigerator so that you'll see it when you're hungry.

NUTRITION INFORMATION:

5+1 = 146 calories, 25g protein, 0g carbs, 4.4g fat

3+1 = 112 calories, 17.5g protein, 0g carbs, 4.4g fat

FISH

My favorite form of protein, fish is tasty, very low calorie, and easy to prepare. Generally speaking, it's best served hot. Cold fish is good—but not exactly an American favorite. Unless it's tuna fish, which I cover here.

A few fish rules: if you're not cooking fresh fish, you'll want to give your frozen portion a chance to thaw slowly. Take out a packet of your frozen fish the night before you plan to use it, and let it thaw in the fridge on a plate. When you're ready to cook, take it out and pat the fish dry. Season it as you wish with herbs or spices, but save any salting for after you cook it.

Roasted Fish

I can see you rolling your eyes. You think this is too hard? Trust me: this is really good! And easy.

INGREDIENTS

6 to 8 ounces tilapia, salmon, trout, bass (farmed), or
    cod fillet
Salt and pepper to taste
2 sprays of olive oil

DIRECTIONS

1. Place a small roasting pan in the oven and preheat to 450°F–500°F.
2. Season the fish on both sides with salt and pepper and any other spices you want to add.
3. Spray a piece of foil with olive oil and set the fish on it.

4. Plop the foil with the fish on the hot pan in the oven. Roast for 8 to 10 minutes. No need to turn the fish; it will roast up nicely on the foil.

5. Take out the fish and let it sit for a minute.

Use to:
- top a huge green salad or plate of roasted veggies
- make a fish sandwich using lettuce "buns" and roasted tomato sauce
- make a great soup by placing the fish in a huge bowl of canned low-salt chicken broth and veggies
- toss bite-size pieces with whole-wheat pasta and roasted tomatoes

NUTRITION INFORMATION (APPROXIMATE PER 6 OUNCES):

Bass: 165 calories, 30g protein, 0g carbs, 4g fat

Cod: 140 calories, 30g protein, 0g carbs, 1.1g fat

Salmon: 202 calories, 35g protein, 0g carbs, 5.8g fat

Tilapia: 198 calories, 32g protein, 0g carbs, 3.4g fat

Trout: 140 calories, 30g protein, 0g carbs, 1.1g fat

"Makes Me Happy" Tuna Salad

INGREDIENTS

¼ cup canned, low-sodium garbanzos, kidney beans, or white beans, drained and rinsed

¼ cup finely diced onion

¼ cup diced tomato

1 tablespoon chopped fresh parsley or basil

1 teaspoon olive oil

2 tablespoons freshly squeezed lemon juice

Pinch of salt

Pinch of freshly ground black pepper

2 large hard-boiled egg whites, sliced

4 to 6 ounces canned water-packed tuna (no salt added), drained

DIRECTIONS

1. Combine all the ingredients except the egg and tuna in a bowl. Toss gently.
2. Place the egg slices and tuna on top.
3. Eat. Good for lunch at work. Eliminate onion if your breath becomes a social issue.

NUTRITION INFORMATION:

331 calories, 47g protein, 18g carbs, 6.5g fat

POULTRY

Herb-Roasted Chicken Breast

You'll see in my menus that I often suggest cubed chicken to top salads or to be served with roasted veggies. This is a great recipe for that use. You can also roast the chicken with my mustard sauce (page 186). Either way, this is the chicken breast to prepare each weekend of your first month of skinny eating.

INGREDIENTS

½ tablespoon mixed fresh herbs (marjoram, oregano, parsley, chives, thyme, etc.)

2 teaspoons freshly squeezed lemon juice

1 teaspoon olive oil

5 ounces boneless, skinless chicken breast

DIRECTIONS

1. Preheat the oven to 350°F.
2. In a small bowl, combine the herbs, lemon juice, and oil.
3. Add the chicken and coat with the herb mixture. Place in a baking dish and bake for 12 to 15 minutes, until no longer pink in the center.

NUTRITION INFORMATION:

138 calories, 27g protein, 2.8g carbs, 1.5g fat

Turkey Meatballs

As I said earlier, you're going to be eating a lot of these wonderful turkey meatballs if you follow my menus. Whether you have just a couple of meatballs as a snack or a larger serving for lunch or dinner, wrap them in lettuce instead of in a bun.

Makes 4 servings

Brown rice is a healthy substitute for the usual bread crumbs.

INGREDIENTS

1 pound extra-lean ground turkey

3 garlic cloves, minced

¼ cup finely chopped onion

¼ cup chopped fresh parsley

½ teaspoon kosher salt

½ teaspoon freshly ground black pepper

½ teaspoon dried oregano

1 large egg, beaten

½ cup cooked brown rice, cooled

Olive oil spray

DIRECTIONS

1. Combine all the ingredients except the olive oil in a large mixing bowl and shape into about 30 meatballs 1 inch across.
2. Spray a large nonstick skillet generously with olive oil.
3. Cook the meatballs for 5 to 6 minutes, working in batches if your pan is not large enough to fit them all, occasionally moving them around to brown all sides.

Variation: Once all the meatballs are cooked, add a jar of low-sodium marinara sauce (preferably organic and with minimal sugar) to the pan. Simmer the meatballs in the sauce for 20 minutes. These sauced meatballs are great by themselves or served over quinoa, farro, or whole-wheat pasta at lunch, or over spaghetti, squash, or other veggies for dinner.

NUTRITION INFORMATION PER SERVING:

213 calories, 24g protein, 8g carbs, 9.6g fat

RED MEAT

The Leanburger

- -

Served with a side salad of mixed greens, ½ sliced tomato, and braised Broccolini (page 181), this makes a really satisfying meal!

INGREDIENTS

4 ounces ground sirloin
1 teaspoon chopped fresh rosemary
2 teaspoons barbecue sauce
Cracked black pepper

DIRECTIONS
1. Heat a small skillet over medium heat.
2. Place the meat in a bowl and mix in all ingredients with your hands. Form a patty and sear in the skillet for at least 2 minutes on each side.
3. Serve with a side salad of 2 cups mixed greens, ½ sliced tomato, and braised Broccolini (page 181).

NUTRITION INFORMATION (BURGER ONLY):

247 calories, 40g protein, 3.2g carbs, 9g fat

BEANS

My Signature No-Oil Hummus

Makes 6 servings; serving size approximately ⅓ cup

INGREDIENTS

2 tablespoons freshly squeezed lemon juice

¼ teaspoon salt

1 15.5-ounce low-sodium can garbanzo beans, drained and rinsed

½ garlic clove, cut into a few smaller pieces

¼ cup low-sodium veggie broth (or water) to thin

DIRECTIONS

1. Place all ingredients in a food processor; process until smooth.
2. Refrigerate in an airtight container for up to 5 days.

NUTRITION INFORMATION PER SERVING:

97.5 calories, 4g protein, 18.7g carbs, 1g fat

VEGETABLES

We come now to the food most of you haven't exactly been gulping down over the past few years; if you had, you would likely be in better shape and less interested in losing weight.

You'll see that we're using a lot of roasting again. I urge you to experiment with the method. We'll also be stir-frying. More pounds have been lost on *TBL* using my dinner version stir-fry recipe than any other dish. If it worked for Olivia (Season 11 winner), it will work for you. Of course, most veggies can also be eaten raw or sautéed—the point is to get more of them into you.

Standard Dinner Salad

Go crazy here with the veg! The more colorful, the more enriched.

INGREDIENTS

2 cups mixed greens

¼ cup each of 4 different vegetables

DIRECTIONS

Pair this salad with any of the roasted proteins mentioned in this book and drizzle with one of my vinaigrettes!

NUTRITION INFORMATION:

Approximately 51 calories, 2g protein, 10g carbs, .5g fat

Bob's Cobb

INGREDIENTS

Harpersized portions of spinach, lettuce, and arugula (i.e., as much
   as you want!)

Harpersized portions of shredded carrots and chopped tomatoes

Pinch (½ ounce) of grated cheddar cheese

3 large hard-boiled egg whites, sliced

1 cup cubed (½-inch dice) chicken

Balsamic Dressing (page 182)

DIRECTIONS

Toss the greens, carrots, and tomatoes together in a large bowl. Top
with the cheese, egg whites, and chicken, and drizzle with dressing.

NUTRITION INFORMATION:

The only calories you need to think about here are those that come
from protein—if you add it—and your chosen dressing. Count those,
but have all the veggies listed here that you want!

My Signature Stir-Fry

Makes 4 servings

With or without adding tofu, this can be your go-to lunch (with the quinoa) or dinner (without the quinoa) recipe for your meatless day (Rule 12). You can add chicken breast or shrimp (1 pound, skinless) to the pan and voilà—this core vegetable recipe instantly becomes a poultry dish!

INGREDIENTS

Olive oil spray

6 to 10 shiitake mushrooms

At least 1 pound assorted vegetables, sliced (try this combo: broccoli, carrots, baby corn, asparagus, snow peas, jicama or water chestnuts, and bean sprouts)

3 garlic cloves, minced

¼ cup raw cashews

2 tablespoons diced jalapeños

1 teaspoon red pepper flakes

1 tablespoon freshly squeezed lime juice

2 cups cooked quinoa

DIRECTIONS

1. Spray a large skillet with olive oil and heat over medium-high heat.
2. Add the mushrooms and sauté for 4 minutes.
3. Toss in the rest of the veggies, the garlic, cashews, jalapeños, and red pepper flakes. Cook for about 5 minutes, stirring occasionally.
4. When the veggies are tender, toss with lime juice.
5. Top the cooked quinoa with the veggies.

LUNCH VERSION NUTRITION INFORMATION PER SERVING WITHOUT CHICKEN:

257 calories, 11g protein, 40g carbs, 7g fat

LUNCH VERSION NUTRITION INFORMATION PER SERVING WITH
CHICKEN:

  382 calories, 37g protein, 40g carbs, 9g fat

DINNER VERSION NUTRITION INFORMATION PER SERVING
WITHOUT CHICKEN:

  76 calories, 3g protein, 8g carbs, 4g fat

DINNER VERSION NUTRITION INFORMATION PER SERVING WITH
CHICKEN:

  201 calories, 29g protein, 9g carbs, 6g fat

> You'll see in my Menus that I distinguish between the lunch and dinner
> versions of this recipe. To be clear: the lunch version means you can
> include the quinoa, but no quinoa for dinner. (No carbs after lunch,
> remember?)

Roasted Yam Hashbrowns

Makes one serving

INGREDIENTS

1 cup cubed (½-inch dice) sweet potatoes
Pinch of salt
Freshly ground black pepper
1 teaspoon your favorite dried herb
3 sprays olive oil

DIRECTIONS

1. Preheat the oven to 400°F.
2. Put the sweet potatoes in a bowl and season with salt and pepper and the herb of your choice. Spray with olive oil and toss to coat, then place on a sheet of aluminum foil or a cookie sheet.
3. Roast for 30 minutes or until soft when probed with the tip of a knife.

NUTRITION INFORMATION:

158 calories, 2g protein, 37g carbs, .2g fat

Roasted Tomatoes

Makes 4 servings

INGREDIENTS

3 pounds ripe tomatoes, cores removed

1 whole head garlic, cut in half lengthwise and coated with olive oil
spray

1 tablespoon olive oil

Pinch of salt and freshly ground black pepper

1 tablespoon chopped fresh herbs

DIRECTIONS

1. Preheat the oven to 450°F.
2. Toss everything together except the herbs.
3. Place the ingredients in a roasting pan, cover with foil, and roast
   for 1 hour and 15 minutes.
4. Remove and let cool. Squish the garlic from the skin and combine with the tomatoes and fresh herbs.

Use to:

- blend into a soup
- serve as a sauce or condiment
- combine with chicken and more veggies for a complete meal

NUTRITION INFORMATION PER SERVING:

101 calories, 3g protein, 16g carbs, 5g fat

Roasted Eggplant

Makes 4 servings

INGREDIENTS
2 pounds eggplant, cubed
Olive oil spray
2 tablespoons minced fresh herbs

DIRECTIONS
1. Preheat the oven to 450°F.
2. Put the eggplant in a large bowl, spray with olive oil, and toss to coat.
3. Place the eggplant in a single layer in a roasting pan and roast for 45 minutes, stirring every 15 minutes.
4. Remove and toss with fresh herbs.

Use to:
- combine with roasted tomatoes (see preceding recipe) to make a ratatouille, or veggie stew
- blend into a puree to serve with meats or as a dip for snacks
- serve on its own as a cold salad using mint, a pinch of brown sugar, and lemon to jazz it up

NUTRITION INFORMATION PER SERVING:
59 calories, 2.5g protein, 14g carbs, .4g fat

Grilled Asparagus

Makes 4 servings

INGREDIENTS

1 pound (1 bunch) asparagus spears
Olive oil spray
½ tablespoon your favorite blend of dry herbs
Pinch of salt
Freshly ground black pepper

DIRECTIONS

1. Preheat your grill or broiler.
2. Trim woody stems from the asparagus. Spray the spears with oil.
3. Place the asparagus on the grill or under the broiler for about 5 minutes, turning occasionally until tender and slightly charred.
4. Toss with the herbs, salt, and pepper.

Use for:

- a lunch salad, topped with diced hard-boiled egg whites, some lemon or mustard, and a few pistachios
- an omelet filling
- a side dish for fish or poultry

NUTRITION INFORMATION PER SERVING:

17 calories, 1.5g protein, 3g carbs, .5g fat

Roasted Cauliflower

Makes 4 servings

INGREDIENTS

1 large head of cauliflower (or 1 bag of pre-separated florets)
Olive oil spray
Salt and freshly ground black pepper
1 tablespoon grated parmesan cheese
Red pepper flakes to taste

DIRECTIONS

1. Preheat the oven to 450°F. Bring a large pot of water to a boil.
2. Separate the head into large florets and plunge them into boiling water for 3 minutes, or until cooked al dente.
3. Drain, dry, and place in an ovenproof pan.
4. Spray with olive oil, then add salt and pepper to taste.
5. Roast for 10 to 15 minutes, until the tops begin to brown.
6. Sprinkle with parmesan and pepper flakes, cook another 2 minutes, and serve.

Use to:
• accompany steak or fish dinners
• mash as a potato substitute
• puree with a few tablespoons milk as a bed for roast chicken breast
• puree with low-salt chicken broth for soup

NUTRITION INFORMATION PER SERVING:
58 calories, 4.7g protein, 11g carbs, .8g fat

Braised Broccoli or Rapini

Makes 4 servings

INGREDIENTS
1 large head of broccoli or 1 bunch of rapini
1 teaspoon olive oil
2 garlic cloves, sliced
Salt and freshly ground black pepper

DIRECTIONS
1. Bring a large pot of water to a boil.
2. Separate the broccoli into small florets. If using rapini, trim the woody ends and cut into 2- to 3-inch lengths.
3. Plunge the broccoli or rapini into boiling water for 3 minutes. Drain in a colander.
4. In a large frying pan, heat the oil with the garlic, then add the broccoli or rapini and stir-fry for 3 minutes.
5. Season to taste with salt and pepper.

Use to:
- stuff omelets
- puree with low-salt canned broth for a healthy and hearty green soup
- toss with whole-wheat pasta or farro

NUTRITION INFORMATION PER SERVING:
54 calories, 4.6g protein, 8g carbs, 1.7g fat

DRESSINGS/SAUCES

Balsamic Dressing

Makes 1 Serving

INGREDIENTS

1 tablespoon balsamic vinegar

1 teaspoon Dijon mustard

2 teaspoons freshly squeezed lemon juice

DIRECTIONS

Whisk ingredients together and drizzle over a salad or roasted vegetables 5 minutes before taking them out of the oven.

NUTRITION INFORMATION:

20 calories, .1g protein, 4.6 carbs, 0g fat

Chili Dressing

INGREDIENTS

1 teaspoon finely chopped green onions (scallions)

1 tablespoon rice wine vinegar

½ teaspoon Bragg Liquid Aminos

⅛ teaspoon minced garlic

⅛ teaspoon minced fresh ginger

Pinch of red pepper flakes

DIRECTIONS

Whisk ingredients together and drizzle over a mixed greens salad.

NUTRITION INFORMATION:

3 calories, .5g protein, .5 carbs, 0g fat

Though this dressing is incredibly low in calories, the Bragg Liquid Aminos ups the sodium content. If you are doubling or tripling the ingredients to make a bigger batch of dressing, just be aware of the sodium level—and don't use more than 1 serving at a time.

Mustard Vinaigrette

INGREDIENTS

1 tablespoon white wine vinegar

2 teaspoons Dijon mustard

1 teaspoon agave

DIRECTIONS

Whisk ingredients together and drizzle over a salad or roasted vegetables 5 minutes before taking them out of the oven.

NUTRITION INFORMATION:

38 calories, 0g protein, 7g carbs, 0g fat

Pesto

- -

Makes 4 servings

INGREDIENTS

   1 cup chopped fresh basil
   1 tablespoon grated parmesan cheese
   1 garlic clove
   ½ tablespoon freshly squeezed lemon juice
   ¼ cup low-sodium vegetable broth
   2 tablespoons chopped walnuts, cashews, or pine nuts

DIRECTIONS

Blend all ingredients in a food processor. Store in the refrigerator up
to 5 days.

NUTRITION INFORMATION PER SERVING:

   26 calories, 1.1g protein, 1.8 carbs, 1.8g fat

Mustard Sauce

INGREDIENTS

    2 tablespoons nonfat Greek yogurt

    2 teaspoons Dijon mustard

    1 teaspoon agave

    ½ teaspoon minced garlic

DIRECTIONS

Mix ingredients in a small bowl. Use to top roasted chicken, steak, or pork.

NUTRITION INFORMATION:

    45 calories, 2g protein, 5.6g carbs, 0g fat

THREE CORE EXTRAS

The Skinny Shake

INGREDIENTS

1½ cups seasonal berries (strawberries, blueberries, blackberries,
etc.)

1 cup nonfat Greek yogurt

12 ounces water or almond milk (I use 6 ounces of each, but see
which you prefer)

DIRECTIONS

Whirl all ingredients in a blender and enjoy!

NUTRITION INFORMATION (WITH ALMOND MILK):

319 calories, 16g protein, 46g carbs, 9g fat

My Mean, Green Drink Meal Replacement

Makes 1 meal replacement or 2 midmorning power boosts

INGREDIENTS

2 tablespoons protein powder (50 calories)

1 cup chopped fresh kale (30 calories)

1 cup frozen spinach (30 calories)

½ cup blueberries (35 calories)

½ small banana (40 calories)

½ cup frozen pineapple (45 calories)

20 ounces water

DIRECTIONS

Place all ingredients in a blender and blend until combined.

NUTRITION INFORMATION:

14g fiber, 340 calories!

Your Own Broth

Broth is the basis of soup—all kinds of soup—and is a perfect Skinny Rules food. It's low in calories, high in nutrients, versatile, and easy to use. On top of that, it will help you feel full because it takes up a lot of space in your stomach. You can buy all kinds of low-salt canned chicken broth, which is perfectly fine. Or you can make your own. For chicken broth:

1. Put a whole uncooked chicken in a big pot and fill with water to the top of the bird.
2. Bring to a boil, skim that weird stuff off the top, and simmer for 4 hours.
3. Take the chicken out of the pot, let cool, and you've got a great broth. As for the bird itself, shred the meat: you can then put it back in whatever soup you are making or use it for sandwiches and salads.

My favorite broth is roasted-tomato broth, which can not only be used for soup, but also for cooking fish (heat a couple cups in a pan; add fish and cook for no more than 10 minutes). It's easy and worth learning. To make it:

1. Preheat the oven to 450°F.
2. Put a bunch of whole tomatoes in a large roasting pan and pop the pan in the oven for 1 hour or until the tomatoes have collapsed and shriveled down.
3. Remove, let the tomatoes cool, then blend to your desired consistency. Thin is best for broth and cooking; thick is good as a catsup-like condiment for turkey burgers.

MORE SKINNY WAY RECIPES

Remember when I said no lime Jell-O omega-3 parfaits? I've decided to spare you those, but I *do* want to give you some recipes you can use to broaden your meal choices. Here are some of my favorites, organized under breakfast, lunch, and dinner. I suggest first trying a few breakfast recipes, perhaps on a Saturday or Sunday morning, when you've got a little time and when you might have an appreciative and hungry audience.

BREAKFAST OPTIONS

B.E.S.T. Breakfast Sandwich

INGREDIENTS

1 ounce (3 pieces) low-sodium turkey bacon

Nonstick cooking spray

3 large egg whites, beaten

2 slices whole-grain bread

½ cup raw spinach, either baby spinach or whole-leaf with stems removed

1 thick slice tomato

DIRECTIONS

1. Cook the bacon according to package instructions. Set aside.
2. Spray a skillet with nonstick cooking spray. Heat over medium heat.
3. Add the egg whites. Scramble.
4. Meanwhile, toast the bread.
5. Place the spinach on 1 slice of toast, layer the tomato, scrambled eggs, and bacon, and top with the other slice of toast. Slice in half on the diagonal.

NUTRITION INFORMATION:

420 calories, 26g protein, 49g carbs, 13g fat

Green Eggs and "Ham"

INGREDIENTS

Nonstick cooking spray

2 thin slices low-sodium turkey bacon

1 teaspoon extra virgin olive oil

½ tablespoon finely chopped fresh basil

½ tablespoon finely chopped fresh parsley

½ cup chopped fresh spinach

5/3+1 Omelet mixture (page 162)

2 teaspoons grated parmesan cheese

1 slice whole-grain bread, toasted

DIRECTIONS

1. Spray a skillet with nonstick cooking spray and heat over medium heat.

2. Add the bacon and crisp for approximately 2 minutes on each side.

3. Remove the bacon, crumble, and set aside. Wipe the inside of the skillet with a paper towel.

4. Pour the olive oil into the skillet, then add the basil, parsley, and spinach. Cook for a few minutes, allowing the spinach to wilt a little. Pour the egg mixture over the greens and scramble.

5. When the eggs are cooked, top with the crumbled bacon, sprinkle with the parmesan, and serve with the toast.

NUTRITION INFORMATION:

5+1 = 272 calories, 29g protein, 15g carbs, 8.4g fat

3+1 = 236 calories, 22g protein, 15g carbs, 8.4g fat

Fresh Herb Omelet

INGREDIENTS

Nonstick cooking spray

5/3+1 Omelet mixture (page 162)

1 teaspoon chopped fresh chives

1 teaspoon chopped fresh parsley

1 teaspoon chopped fresh basil

1 teaspoon chopped fresh oregano

DIRECTIONS

1. Spray a skillet with nonstick cooking spray and heat over medium heat.
2. Mix the eggs with the herbs.
3. Pour the eggs into the skillet and cook slowly, lifting up the edges occasionally and letting the liquid run underneath.
4. After 3 minutes, flip the omelet.
5. Let cook for 2 minutes, then slide onto a plate.

NUTRITION INFORMATION:

5+1 = 146 calories, 25g protein, 0g carbs, 4.4g fat

3+1 = 112 calories, 17.5g protein, 0g carbs, 4.4g fat

Mushroom Asparagus Scramble

INGREDIENTS

Nonstick cooking spray

4 cremini mushrooms, chopped

3 asparagus spears, woody stems trimmed, sliced into ¼-inch
rounds

½ tablespoon chopped shallot

1 teaspoon Bragg Liquid Aminos

5/3+1 Omelet mixture (page 162)

DIRECTIONS

1. Spray a skillet with nonstick cooking spray.
2. Heat the skillet over medium heat. Add the mushrooms, asparagus, and shallot and cook for about 4 minutes.
3. Drizzle in the Bragg Liquid Aminos and stir until absorbed.
4. Add the eggs and scramble until done.

NUTRITION INFORMATION:

5+1 = 164 calories, 27g protein, 3.6g carbs, 4.6g fat

3+1 = 131 calories, 20.5g protein, 3.6g carbs, 4.6g fat

Italian Egg Sandwich

INGREDIENTS

Nonstick cooking spray

5/3+1 Omelet mixture (page 162)

½ tablespoon chopped fresh basil

1 tablespoon grated parmesan cheese

¼ cup chopped red bell pepper

½ small plum tomato, chopped

1 whole-wheat English muffin

DIRECTIONS

1. Spray a skillet with nonstick cooking spray.
2. Mix the eggs with the basil and parmesan. Set aside.
3. Heat the skillet over medium heat. Add the pepper and tomato and cook for about 4 minutes.
4. Add the egg mixture and scramble until done.
5. While the eggs are cooking, toast the English muffin. Spoon the eggs over the muffin.

NUTRITION INFORMATION:

5+1 = 317 calories, 33g protein, 30g carbs, 7.5g fat

3+1 = 283 calories, 26g protein, 30g carbs, 7.5g fat

Huevos Rancheros

INGREDIENTS

2 6-inch whole-wheat tortillas

Nonstick cooking spray

5/3+1 Omelet mixture (page 162)

¼ cup low- or no-sodium canned black beans, drained and rinsed

¼ cup green salsa

¼ avocado, sliced

DIRECTIONS

1. Toast the tortillas in a toaster oven or regular oven on 350°F for 5 minutes, until crisp.
2. Spray a skillet with nonstick cooking spray and heat over medium heat.
3. Add the eggs and scramble.
4. Set the eggs on the tortillas.
5. Add the beans and salsa to the pan and heat through.
6. Top the tortillas and eggs with beans and salsa. Add avocado and enjoy.

NUTRITION INFORMATION:

5+1 = 469 calories, 43g protein, 43g carbs, 18g fat

3+1 = 435 calories, 35g protein, 43g carbs, 18g fat

B.L.T. Scramble

INGREDIENTS

Nonstick cooking spray

2 slices low-sodium turkey bacon

3 large egg whites

1 tomato, diced

¼ avocado, thinly sliced

1 slice whole-grain bread, toasted

DIRECTIONS

1. Spray a skillet with nonstick cooking spray and heat over medium heat.
2. Add the bacon and crisp for about 2 minutes on each side.
3. Remove the bacon from the skillet, let cool, then crumble.
4. Wipe the inside of the skillet with a paper towel. Scramble the egg whites in the skillet with the tomato and crumbled bacon.
5. Transfer to a plate, top with avocado, and serve with the toast.

NUTRITION INFORMATION:

349 calories, 21g protein, 29g carbs, 16g fat

Peppery Breakfast Pita

Arugula has a wonderful peppery flavor and really perks up the standard omelet/scramble ingredients here.

INGREDIENTS
    Nonstick cooking spray
    ½ cup chopped arugula
    5/3+1 Omelet mixture (page 162)
    1 ounce mozzarella cheese
    1 whole-wheat medium pita, warmed

DIRECTIONS
1. Spray a skillet with nonstick cooking spray and heat over medium heat.
2. Add the arugula and cook, stirring, until wilted, 2 to 3 minutes.
3. Add the eggs and cheese. Scramble.
4. Stuff the warmed pita and enjoy.

NUTRITION INFORMATION:
    5+1 = 404 calories, 38g protein, 36g carbs, 11.4g fat
    3+1 = 370 calories, 30.5g protein, 36g carbs, 11.4g fat

Caprese Breakfast Wrap

INGREDIENTS

Nonstick cooking spray

5/3+1 Omelet mixture (page 162)

1 tablespoon chopped fresh basil

1 10-inch whole-wheat tortilla

1 small plum tomato, sliced

2 ounces mozzarella cheese

DIRECTIONS

1. Spray a skillet with nonstick cooking spray and heat over medium heat.
2. Add the eggs and basil. Scramble until done.
3. Place in the tortilla and top with the tomato and mozzarella. Wrap like a burrito.

NUTRITION INFORMATION:

288 calories, 18g protein, 28g carbs, 12g fat

Sweet Potato and Herb Frittata

INGREDIENTS

Olive oil spray

1 tablespoon finely chopped red onion

¼ cup thinly sliced red bell pepper

¼ cup shredded sweet potato

5/3+1 Omelet mixture (page 162)

1 tablespoon chopped fresh basil

1 teaspoon finely chopped fresh rosemary

DIRECTIONS

1. Turn on the broiler. While it heats, set a medium skillet on the stove and heat on medium-high. Spray the skillet with olive oil.

2. Place the onion, pepper, and sweet potato in the skillet and sauté for 5 minutes. Turn the heat to low.

3. Pour the eggs, basil, and rosemary over the vegetables and let the mixture cook slowly, lifting up the edges occasionally to check that the frittata is not burning.

4. When the eggs appear almost done, place the skillet under the broiler. Check after a minute: the top should just be beginning to brown.

5. Remove from the broiler, and let sit for a few minutes; then slide the frittata onto a plate. Eat immediately.

NUTRITION INFORMATION:

5+1 = 203 calories, 27g protein, 13g carbs, 4.6g fat

3+1 = 169 calories, 19g protein, 13g carbs, 4.6g fat

Spring Vegetable Omelet

INGREDIENTS
Nonstick cooking spray

5/3+1 Omelet mixture (page 162)

¼ cup diced tomatoes

¼ cup diced zucchini

¼ cup diced red bell pepper

½ cup chopped fresh spinach

1 whole-grain English muffin or slice of whole-grain bread, toasted

DIRECTIONS
1. Spray a medium skillet with nonstick cooking spray. Preheat over medium heat.
2. Combine the eggs and vegetables in a medium bowl.
3. Pour the mixture into the skillet and cook over medium heat for several minutes, occasionally lifting up edges to let the egg run underneath.
4. Fold and flatten with a spatula.
5. Flip once and continue to cook for another minute.
6. Serve with the toasted whole-grain English muffin.

NUTRITION INFORMATION:
5+1 = 308 calories, 32g protein, 33g carbs, 6g fat

3+1 = 274 calories, 24g protein, 33g carbs, 6g fat

Breakfast Quesadilla

INGREDIENTS

Nonstick cooking spray

¼ cup chopped bell pepper

¼ cup finely chopped fresh spinach

¼ cup chopped tomato

⅛ teaspoon cumin

⅛ teaspoon chili powder

5/3+1 Omelet mixture (page 162)

2 6-inch whole-wheat tortillas

¼ avocado, sliced

Dash of freshly ground black pepper

DIRECTIONS

1. Preheat the oven to 350°F. Spray a skillet with nonstick cooking spray and heat over medium heat.
2. Add the bell pepper, spinach, tomato, cumin, and chili powder. Sauté for 2 minutes.
3. Add the eggs and scramble.
4. Place the tortillas on a baking sheet. Top one tortilla with the egg mixture, add the avocado and pepper, and cover with the second tortilla.
5. Press down gently and place in the oven for 10 minutes. (You can also cook the quesadilla in a large skillet set over medium heat and sprayed with olive oil; press it down with a spatula.)
6. Cut into triangles and enjoy.

NUTRITION INFORMATION:

5+1 = 399 calories, 31g protein, 33g carbs, 16.4g fat

3+1 = 357 calories, 23g protein, 33g carbs, 16.4g fat

Berry Quinoa Breakfast Cereal

INGREDIENTS
¼ cup uncooked quinoa, rinsed under cold water and drained

¼ cup almond milk

½ cup water

½ tablespoon ground flax seed

¼ teaspoon cinnamon

½ cup mixed berries

DIRECTIONS
1. Combine the quinoa, milk, and water in a saucepan. Heat over high heat until it comes to a boil.
2. Reduce the heat to medium-low, cover, and simmer for about 15 minutes, until the quinoa is fluffy and the liquid is mostly absorbed.
3. Stir in flax seed, cinnamon, and berries.

NUTRITION INFORMATION:
216 calories, 8g protein, 36g carbs, 5g fat

Fall Pumpkin Oatmeal

INGREDIENTS

½ cup rolled oats

¼ cup almond or skim milk

½ cup water

¼ teaspoon cinnamon

¼ teaspoon nutmeg

¼ cup canned pumpkin puree

½ tablespoon ground flax seed

1 tablespoon chopped nuts (walnuts, pecans, or almonds)

DIRECTIONS

1. Combine the oats, milk, water, cinnamon, and nutmeg in a small saucepan. Bring to a slow simmer.
2. Add the pumpkin puree, flax seed, and nuts.
3. Stir to combine and simmer until the oatmeal is done, 3 to 4 minutes.

NUTRITION INFORMATION:

255 calories, 9g protein, 34g carbs, 10g fat

Apple 'n' Nut Oatmeal

INGREDIENTS

½ cup rolled oats

¼ cup water

¼ cup almond milk

½ apple, cubed

12 raw almonds, finely chopped

¼ teaspoon cinnamon

Pinch of nutmeg

1 tablespoon ground flax seed

DIRECTIONS

1. Combine the oats, water, almond milk, and apple in a small saucepan and simmer over low heat for 5 minutes.
2. Stir in the almonds, cinnamon, nutmeg, and flax seed.

NUTRITION INFORMATION:

212 calories, 8g protein, 19g carbs, 12g fat

Banana-Blueberry Protein Pancakes

INGREDIENTS

Nonstick cooking spray

½ cup rolled oats

¼ cup fat-free ricotta

4 large egg whites

½ banana

⅛ teaspoon baking powder

½ teaspoon vanilla extract

½ cup blueberries

DIRECTIONS

1. Spray a large skillet or griddle with nonstick cooking spray and heat over medium heat.
2. Mix all ingredients together well except the blueberries.
3. Fold the blueberries into the batter.
4. When the skillet is hot (a drop of batter should sizzle immediately), pour 4 separate dollops of batter to form pancakes.
5. Cook over medium heat for about 90 seconds per side, flipping once.

NUTRITION INFORMATION:

380 calories, 38g protein, 51g carbs, 9.2g fat

Banana-Nut Pancakes

INGREDIENTS

Nonstick cooking spray

4 large egg whites

½ cup rolled oats

¼ cup unsweetened applesauce

½ teaspoon cinnamon

½ teaspoon vanilla extract

⅛ teaspoon baking powder

1 banana, sliced

2 tablespoons chopped pecans

DIRECTIONS

1. Spray a skillet or griddle with nonstick cooking spray; heat over medium heat.
2. Put all ingredients except the banana and pecans in a food processor and blend to make the batter.
3. Fold in the banana and pecans.
4. Pour the batter into the skillet, forming a single large pancake.
5. Cook over medium heat for 60 to 90 seconds per side.

NUTRITION INFORMATION:

397 calories, 24g protein, 34g carbs, 19g fat

Banana-Nut Cinnamon Muffins

Makes 4 muffins, 2 servings

INGREDIENTS

1 small extra-ripe banana
2 teaspoons cinnamon
8 large egg whites
1 cup rolled oats
½ cup unsweetened applesauce
2 tablespoons chopped walnuts

DIRECTIONS

1. Preheat the oven to 350°F.
2. Mash the banana in a small bowl with a fork.
3. Mix all ingredients except the walnuts in a food processor or blender.
4. Fold the walnuts into the batter.
5. Line 4 of the cups in a 6-cup muffin pan with paper liners. Divide the mixture among the lined muffin cups.
6. Bake for 20 to 25 minutes or until done. (A toothpick inserted in the center should come out clean.)

NUTRITION INFORMATION PER SERVING:

343 calories, 24g protein, 47g carbs, 7.6g fat

Sweet Potato and Oat Pancakes with Warmed Berries

Makes 1 large pancake or 2 or 3 smaller pancakes

INGREDIENTS

1 medium sweet potato, cooked, cooled, and diced

¼ cup rolled oats

4 large egg whites

¼ teaspoon vanilla extract

½ teaspoon cinnamon

⅛ teaspoon nutmeg

½ tablespoon ground flax seed

¼ cup blackberries

2 tablespoons water

Nonstick cooking spray

DIRECTIONS

1. Combine the sweet potato, oats, egg whites, vanilla, spices, and flax seed in a blender or food processor. Blend until smooth.
2. Spray a large skillet or griddle with nonstick cooking spray. Heat over medium heat.
3. Put the berries and water in a small pot and simmer over low heat for 5 minutes. Mash with a fork.
4. Pour the batter into the skillet, forming a single large pancake or several smaller ones.
5. Cook for 1½ to 2 minutes per side, flipping once.
6. Serve the pancakes topped with warm berry sauce.

NUTRITION INFORMATION:

253 calories, 21g protein, 36g carbs, 3g fat

Mango and Blueberry Parfait

INGREDIENTS

6 ounces nonfat Greek yogurt

½ cup diced mango

½ cup blueberries

1 tablespoon pumpkin seeds

DIRECTIONS

1. Spoon half the yogurt into a dish. Top with half the fruit and pumpkin seeds.
2. Top with the rest of the yogurt, fruit, and seeds.

NUTRITION INFORMATION:

203 calories, 7g protein, 43g carbs, 1.5g fat

Strawberry-Banana Smoothie

INGREDIENTS

  6 ounces nonfat Greek yogurt

  ½ frozen banana (if fresh, add ice)

  1 cup sliced strawberries

  ½ cup orange juice with pulp

DIRECTIONS

1. Put all ingredients in a blender and blend to the desired consistency.

2. Pour into a tall glass.

NUTRITION INFORMATION:

  235 calories, 7.5g protein, 52g carbs, 1.3g fat

Apple Berry Shake

INGREDIENTS

½ apple

1 cup chopped kale

½ cup mixed berries

1 tablespoon ground flax seed

1 cup almond milk

¼ cup ice

DIRECTIONS

Blend all ingredients in a blender until smooth.

NUTRITION INFORMATION:

337 calories, 9g protein, 42g carbs, 12g fat

LOTS OF LUNCH

Here are some of my favorite lunch recipes. They're easy to fix without tons of prep, and once you try a few, you'll see that your midday meals need never be boring or unsatisfying.

Southwestern Chicken with Kale

INGREDIENTS

Olive oil spray

¼ onion, diced

1 teaspoon dried oregano

1 teaspoon ground cumin

1 teaspoon chili powder

¼ cup uncooked quinoa

½ cup low-sodium vegetable broth

2 cups finely chopped kale

¼ cup low-sodium canned black beans, drained and rinsed

½ tomato, diced

3 ounces cooked chicken, cubed

DIRECTIONS

1. Heat a saucepan over medium-high heat. Coat with olive oil, add the onion, and sauté until mostly translucent and tender.
2. Add the spices and quinoa. Toast for 2 minutes.
3. Pour in the broth, lower the heat, and simmer for 10 to 15 minutes, or until the quinoa is tender and the liquid is absorbed.
4. Stir in the kale and cook until wilted, about 2 minutes.
5. Fold in the beans, tomato, and chicken and heat through.

NUTRITION INFORMATION:

232 calories, 29g protein, 22g carbs, 3.5g fat

Chipotle Turkey Tacos

INGREDIENTS

1 tablespoon olive oil

¼ yellow onion, chopped

¼ red bell pepper, chopped

3 ounces extra-lean ground turkey

1 chipotle pepper in adobo (canned), seeded and chopped

¼ teaspoon ground cumin

¼ teaspoon red pepper flakes

¼ teaspoon freshly ground black pepper

½ tomato, diced

2 6-inch whole-wheat or whole-grain tortillas

½ cup chopped lettuce

Salsa (optional)

DIRECTIONS

1. Heat the olive oil in a skillet over medium heat.
2. Add the onion and pepper. Sauté for 5 minutes until tender.
3. Add the turkey, chipotle, cumin, red and black pepper, and to-mato. Cook, stirring occasionally, until done (the turkey is no longer pink).
4. Divide the mixture evenly between 2 tortillas. Top with lettuce and salsa, if desired.

NUTRITION INFORMATION:

340 calories, 32g protein, 37g carbs, 11g fat

Ahi Tacos with Mango Salad

INGREDIENTS

4 ounces ahi tuna fillet

Olive oil spray

Salt and freshly ground black pepper

¼ cup cubed mango

¼ avocado, cubed

1 tablespoon finely minced red onion

2 teaspoons finely chopped fresh cilantro

1 teaspoon freshly squeezed lime juice

2 6-inch whole-wheat or whole-grain tortillas

½ cup shredded red leaf lettuce or Napa cabbage

Salsa (optional)

DIRECTIONS

1. Heat a skillet for 1 or 2 minutes, until the surface is scalding hot. Meanwhile, coat the tuna with a little olive oil spray and season with a hint of salt and black pepper.

2. Place the tuna on the hot skillet for about 45 seconds; it's going to be noisy.

3. Flip the tuna and cook the other side for 45 seconds to 1 minute. (If you don't like your tuna rare in the middle, cook for 30 seconds longer.) Remove from the pan, set aside, and cut into thin slices.

4. In a small bowl, lightly toss the mango, avocado, onion, cilantro, and lime juice.

5. Distribute half of the tuna on each tortilla. Add the mango-avocado mixture. Top with lettuce or cabbage and salsa, if desired.

NUTRITION INFORMATION:

466 calories, 50g protein, 41g carbs, 15g fat

Turkey and Spinach Bolognese

INGREDIENTS

¼ cup uncooked whole-wheat or whole-grain pasta (½ cup cooked)

Olive oil spray

¼ yellow onion, chopped

1 garlic clove, finely chopped

4 ounces lean ground turkey

1 teaspoon Italian seasoning

¼ cup low-sodium chicken broth

½ cup low-sodium spaghetti sauce

1 cup chopped fresh spinach

DIRECTIONS

1. Cook the pasta according to package directions. Drain.
2. Heat a medium skillet over medium-high heat and spray with olive oil. Add the onion and garlic and sauté for 1 to 2 minutes.
3. Mix in the turkey and Italian seasoning. Cook, stirring occasionally, until done (the turkey is no longer pink).
4. Add the chicken broth and simmer for 4 minutes.
5. Mix in the spaghetti sauce and simmer for 5 minutes.
6. Add the spinach and pasta. Heat for 3 to 5 minutes. (The spinach will wilt down.)

NUTRITION INFORMATION:

271 calories, 27g protein, 24g carbs, 9g fat

Turkey Chili

INGREDIENTS

Olive oil spray

½ small yellow onion, diced

1 garlic clove, minced

½ red bell pepper, diced

½ small zucchini, cubed

4 ounces ground white meat turkey

¼ teaspoon ground cumin

¼ teaspoon chili powder

¼ teaspoon freshly ground black pepper

1 14-ounce can tomatoes, pureed

½ cup low-sodium vegetable broth

2 cups finely chopped kale

DIRECTIONS

1. Spray a skillet with olive oil. Add the onion, garlic, bell pepper and zucchini. Cook for 4 to 5 minutes or until tender.
2. Add the turkey, cumin, chili powder, and black pepper. Cook for an additional 4 minutes.
3. Add the pureed tomatoes and broth.
4. Heat on high, bringing contents almost to a boil and stirring often.
5. Reduce the heat to low, cover, and simmer for 10 minutes. (Add broth or water if the chili gets too thick.)
6. Remove from the heat and stir in the kale until wilted.

NUTRITION INFORMATION:

315 calories, 30g protein, 33g carbs, 9g fat

Garden Turkey Pita

INGREDIENTS

1 teaspoon Dijon mustard

1 tablespoon My Signature No-Oil Hummus (page 170)

1 whole-wheat or whole-grain pita

1 handful of baby spinach

½ tomato, sliced

½ Persian cucumber, sliced on a bias

¼ avocado, sliced

2½ ounces low-sodium turkey breast deli slices

DIRECTIONS

1. Spread the mustard and hummus on the inside of the pita.
2. Add the spinach, tomato, cucumber, avocado, and turkey.

NUTRITION INFORMATION:

332 calories, 16g protein, 39g carbs, 2g fat

Mediterranean Salad with Grilled Chicken

INGREDIENTS

Dressing:

   1 tablespoon red wine vinegar
   1 teaspoon Dijon mustard
   1 teaspoon freshly squeezed lemon juice
   Pinch of dried oregano

Salad:

   3 cups chopped mixed greens
   ½ tomato, chopped
   1 Persian cucumber, chopped
   2 tablespoons crumbled feta cheese
   ¼ cup low-sodium canned garbanzo beans, drained and rinsed
   2 tablespoons sliced kalamata olives
   3 ounces grilled chicken breast, thinly sliced

DIRECTIONS
1. In a small bowl, whisk the dressing ingredients together.
2. Place the mixed greens in a salad bowl.
3. Add the tomato, cucumber, feta, garbanzos, and olives.
4. Drizzle the dressing on top and lightly toss.
5. Top the salad with the chicken.

NUTRITION INFORMATION:
   254 calories, 27g protein, 16g carbs, 8g fat

Fig Salad

INGREDIENTS

Salad:

2 cups mixed greens

2 fresh figs, quartered

5 ounces halibut, broiled

¼ cup canned garbanzo beans, drained and rinsed

1 Persian cucumber, diced

¼ avocado, cubed

1 tablespoon crumbled goat cheese

Dressing:

2 teaspoons white wine vinegar

1 teaspoon freshly squeezed lemon juice

1 teaspoon Dijon mustard

DIRECTIONS

1. Top mixed greens with the figs, halibut, garbanzo beans, cucumber, avocado, and cheese.
2. Combine the dressing ingredients, drizzle over the salad, and toss gently.

NUTRITION INFORMATION:

394 calories, 32g protein, 39g carbs, 12g fat

French Chicken Salad Lettuce Wraps

INGREDIENTS

    3 ounces cooked chicken breast, diced (or 3 ounces cooked tempeh)

    ½ apple, diced

    1 celery stalk, chopped

    2 teaspoons finely minced shallot

    1 teaspoon finely chopped fresh tarragon (or ½ teaspoon dried)

    1 tablespoon chopped raw or toasted walnuts

    1 teaspoon white wine vinegar

    2 tablespoons nonfat Greek yogurt

    3 lettuce leaves (butter leaf or romaine)

DIRECTIONS

1. Combine all ingredients except the lettuce in a bowl and gently mix.
2. Spoon even amounts of the chicken salad into the lettuce leaves.

NUTRITION INFORMATION:

    219 calories, 23g protein, 18g carbs, 6g fat

Tuna Garbanzo Niçoise Salad

INGREDIENTS

Tuna:

1 tablespoon finely minced white onion

½ tablespoon finely minced red onion

1 teaspoon freshly squeezed lemon juice

1 teaspoon Dijon mustard

2 teaspoons white wine vinegar

3 ounces canned water-packed tuna (no salt added), drained

Dash of freshly ground black pepper

Salad:

¼ cup low-sodium canned garbanzo beans, drained and rinsed

1 Persian cucumber, sliced on a bias

3 cups chopped mixed greens

1 large hard-boiled egg, sliced

DIRECTIONS

1. Combine all the tuna ingredients in a small bowl.
2. Combine all the salad ingredients except the egg in a separate bowl.
3. Place the salad mixture on a plate and top with the tuna mixture and sliced egg.

NUTRITION INFORMATION:

303 calories, 32g protein, 32g carbs, 7g fat

Eggplant Pizza Muffins

INGREDIENTS

2 slices eggplant (¼ inch thick)

1 whole-wheat or whole-grain English muffin

1 tablespoon low-sodium marinara sauce

1 tablespoon grated mozzarella cheese

DIRECTIONS

1. Preheat the oven to 350°F.
2. Place the eggplant in a steamer basket set over simmering water and steam the slices until just tender, about 5 minutes.
3. Meanwhile, place the muffin halves on a small baking sheet.
4. When the eggplant is done, place one eggplant slice on each muffin half.
5. Spread marinara sauce over each half and sprinkle the cheese on top.
6. Place in the oven for 5 to 7 minutes or until the cheese is melted.

NUTRITION INFORMATION:

255 calories, 17g protein, 40g carbs, 4g fat

Rancho Fajitas

INGREDIENTS

2 6-inch whole-wheat or
   whole-grain tortillas

1 tablespoon olive oil

¼ onion, sliced

1 garlic clove, minced

½ red bell pepper, sliced into
   strips

½ teaspoon ground cumin

½ teaspoon chili powder

½ teaspoon dried oregano

3 ounces lean sirloin steak (or
   tempeh), sliced into thin strips

½ cup chopped tomatoes

2 cups chopped fresh spinach

½ cup shredded lettuce

1 tablespoon nonfat Greek yogurt

Salsa (optional)

DIRECTIONS

1. Preheat the oven to 350°F. Wrap the tortillas in foil and place in the oven for 3 to 4 minutes to warm. When heated through, place the tortillas on a plate.
2. Meanwhile, pour the oil into a skillet. Heat over medium-high heat.
3. Add the onion, garlic, bell pepper, cumin, chili powder, and oregano; sauté for 1 to 2 minutes or until the onion is tender.
4. Add the steak (or tempeh) to the skillet. Cook for about 2 minutes, until the steak is tender and no longer pink (or tempeh is golden brown).
5. Add the tomatoes and spinach and continue cooking for 3 minutes.
6. When the spinach has wilted and most of the liquid has evaporated, divide the contents evenly among the 2 tortillas.
7. Top with shredded lettuce. Add a dollop of yogurt and salsa, if using, on top.

NUTRITION INFORMATION:

439 calories, 45g protein, 46g carbs, 13g fat

Tuna-Farro-Veggie Salad

INGREDIENTS

½ cup cooked farro, cooled

1 teaspoon chopped fresh oregano (or ½ teaspoon dried)

1 teaspoon chopped fresh parsley (or ½ teaspoon dried)

1 teaspoon Dijon mustard

2 teaspoons white wine vinegar

1 teaspoon freshly squeezed lemon juice

3 ounces canned water-packed tuna (no salt added), drained

2 tablespoons chopped kalamata olives

2 teaspoons drained, rinsed, and chopped capers

½ cup halved cherry tomatoes

¼ cup low-sodium canned white beans (cannellini or navy), drained
    and rinsed

DIRECTIONS

1. In a bowl, mix the farro with the oregano, parsley, mustard, vinegar, and lemon.
2. Lightly toss in chunks of tuna and the olives, capers, cherry tomatoes, and beans.

NUTRITION INFORMATION:

363 calories, 31g protein, 51g carbs, 2g fat

Farro Stir-Fry

INGREDIENTS

Nonstick cooking spray

¼ cup chopped yellow onion

½ carrot, sliced on a bias

4 ounces chicken breast, sliced into strips

½ cup broccoli florets

½ cup sliced zucchini

1 tablespoon Bragg Liquid Aminos

½ tablespoon almond butter

1 teaspoon toasted sesame oil

½ cup cooked farro

DIRECTIONS

1. Spray a skillet with nonstick cooking spray and heat over medium heat.
2. Add the onion and carrot and sauté for 3 to 5 minutes, until tender.
3. Add the chicken and stir. Continue cooking for 3 minutes.
4. Add the broccoli, zucchini, Bragg Liquid Aminos, almond butter, and sesame oil.
5. Cook for 5 more minutes and serve over warm farro.

NUTRITION INFORMATION:

442 calories, 36g protein, 48g carbs, 12g fat

Curried Chicken and Quinoa Salad

INGREDIENTS

3 ounces cooked chicken breast, cooled

¼ teaspoon curry powder

¼ cup nonfat Greek yogurt

¼ cup cooked quinoa

¼ cup chopped apple

½ celery stalk, green parts only, finely chopped

1 tablespoon golden raisins

2 cups chopped fresh spinach

DIRECTIONS

1. In a bowl, mix all the ingredients together except the spinach.
2. Serve the salad over the spinach.

NUTRITION INFORMATION:

283 calories, 27g protein, 39g carbs, 3g fat

Spicy Quinoa Paella

INGREDIENTS

Olive oil spray

¼ onion, chopped

1 garlic clove, crushed

½ red bell pepper, diced

Pinch of red pepper flakes

¼ teaspoon dried oregano

¼ teaspoon ground coriander

½ cup diced zucchini

4 ounces chicken, cubed

¼ cup uncooked quinoa, rinsed and drained

¾ cup low-sodium chicken broth

2 cups chopped fresh spinach

DIRECTIONS

1. Heat a skillet over medium-high heat. Coat with olive oil spray.
2. Sauté the onion, garlic, and bell pepper for 4 to 5 minutes, until tender.
3. Stir in the pepper flakes, oregano, coriander, and zucchini and cook for 2 minutes.
4. Add the chicken and sauté for 3 minutes, stirring occasionally to cook all sides.
5. Add the quinoa and allow it to toast for 2 minutes.
6. Pour in the broth, lower the heat, and cover. Cook for 15 minutes, or until the quinoa is cooked through and the broth is absorbed.
7. Add the spinach and stir in until wilted.

NUTRITION INFORMATION:

363 calories, 5g protein, 45g carbs, 5g fat

Grilled Chicken with Oregano-Mint Quinoa

INGREDIENTS

Olive oil spray

¼ cup finely chopped yellow onion

¼ cup uncooked quinoa, rinsed and drained

½ cup low-sodium chicken broth

1 teaspoon chopped fresh oregano (or ½ teaspoon dried)

1 teaspoon chopped fresh mint

2 teaspoons freshly squeezed lemon juice

2 teaspoons freshly squeezed orange juice

1 teaspoon white wine vinegar

1 Persian cucumber, diced

½ tomato, chopped

3 ounces cooked chicken, cubed

2 cups chopped fresh spinach

DIRECTIONS

1. Heat a saucepan over medium-high heat. Coat with olive oil spray, add the onion, and sauté for 4 minutes.

2. Add the quinoa and toast for 2 minutes. Pour in the broth, lower the heat, and simmer for 10 to 15 minutes, or until the quinoa is cooked through and the broth is absorbed. Cool.

3. Stir in the oregano, mint, lemon juice, orange juice, and vinegar.

4. Toss in the cucumber, tomato, chicken, and spinach.

NUTRITION INFORMATION:

312 calories, 29g protein, 40g carbs, 4.6g fat

Mushroom Barley Soup

INGREDIENTS

Olive oil spray

¼ yellow onion, finely chopped

1 celery stalk, green part only, chopped

½ carrot, chopped

1 bay leaf

4 ounces chicken, cubed

1 teaspoon fresh thyme

5 white button mushrooms, sliced

¼ cup uncooked barley

2 cups low-sodium chicken broth

1 tablespoon minced fresh parsley

DIRECTIONS

1. Heat a skillet over medium-high heat. Spray with olive oil.
2. Add the onion, celery, carrot, and bay leaf. Sauté for 4 to 5 minutes, until the vegetables are tender.
3. Add the chicken, thyme, and mushrooms and cook for 5 more minutes.
4. Add the barley and allow to toast for 2 minutes.
5. Pour in the broth, lower the heat, and simmer for 25 minutes, or until the barley is tender.
6. Garnish with parsley.

NUTRITION INFORMATION:

241 calories, 31g protein, 23g carbs, 3g fat

Hearty Tomato-Basil Soup

INGREDIENTS

Olive oil spray

¼ cup coarsely chopped yellow onion

1 small garlic clove, chopped

¼ cup coarsely chopped carrot

1 bay leaf

¼ teaspoon red pepper flakes

1 cup low-sodium diced canned tomatoes

½ cup low-sodium canned white beans (cannellini, navy, etc.),
   drained and rinsed

1 cup low-sodium chicken broth

1 tablespoon chopped fresh basil

DIRECTIONS

1. Heat a saucepan over medium-high heat and spray with olive oil.
2. Add the onion, garlic, carrot, bay leaf, and red pepper flakes. Sauté for 4 to 5 minutes, until the onion and carrot are tender.
3. Add the tomatoes, beans, and chicken broth. Bring to a boil, then turn the heat to low and simmer for 15 minutes.
4. Remove from the heat and let cool slightly. Remove the bay leaf and add the basil.
5. Pour into a blender or food processor and blend until smooth.
6. Reheat in the same pan and enjoy.

NUTRITION INFORMATION:

197 calories, 11g protein, 36g carbs, 2g fat

Savory Lentil Soup

INGREDIENTS

¼ cup dried lentils

Olive oil spray

¼ cup chopped carrot

2 tablespoons chopped onion

2 tablespoons chopped celery

1 garlic clove, minced

1 bay leaf

½ teaspoon dried thyme

½ tablespoon tomato paste

½ cup cubed peeled sweet potato

1½ cups low-sodium chicken
   broth

Dash of salt and freshly ground
   black pepper

½ tablespoon chopped fresh
   parsley

½ tablespoon grated parmesan
   cheese

DIRECTIONS

1. Rinse and drain the lentils; set aside. Coat a medium pot with olive oil spray.

2. Add the carrot, onion, celery, and garlic to the pot and sauté over medium heat for 5 minutes or until tender.

3. Add the bay leaf, thyme, and tomato paste and stir for 1 minute.

4. Add the lentils and sweet potato and stir for another minute.

5. Add the broth and bring to a boil; then reduce the heat, cover, and simmer for 15 to 20 minutes or until vegetables and lentils are tender. Stir occasionally.

6. Season with salt and pepper to taste. Serve hot with a sprinkling of parsley and parmesan.

NUTRITION INFORMATION:

217 calories, 10g protein, 42g carbs, 2g fat

Pesto Avocado Wrap

INGREDIENTS

1 6-inch whole-wheat or whole-grain tortilla

1 tablespoon Pesto (page 185)

½ cup chopped fresh spinach

3 ounces sliced grilled chicken (or cooked tempeh)

½ cup loosely packed alfalfa sprouts

1 slice tomato, 1½ inches thick, quartered

½ Persian cucumber, sliced

¼ avocado, sliced or cubed

DIRECTIONS

1. Place the tortilla on a plate and spread with the pesto.
2. Place the spinach down the center, then add the chicken or tempeh.
3. Layer the sprouts, tomato, cucumber, and avocado on top.
4. Fold to form a wrap.

NUTRITION INFORMATION:

348 calories, 26g protein, 31g carbs, 15g fat

Open-Faced Mediterranean Veggie Burger

INGREDIENTS

¼ cup rolled oats

¼ red bell pepper, coarsely chopped

¼ red onion, coarsely chopped

¼ cup low-sodium canned garbanzo beans, drained and rinsed

1 large egg white

1 teaspoon garlic powder

1 tablespoon chopped fresh parsley

Nonstick cooking spray

½ whole-wheat or whole-grain English muffin, toasted

1 tomato, sliced

1 tablespoon nonfat Greek yogurt

DIRECTIONS

1. Preheat the oven to 375°F.
2. Put the oats in a food processor, grind until fine, and transfer to a small bowl.
3. Put the pepper and onion in the food processor and pulse to finely dice.
4. Put the garbanzos in a medium bowl and mash with a fork.
5. Add the oats, pepper, and onion to the garbanzos.
6. In a small bowl, combine the egg white, garlic powder, and parsley. Whisk together and pour over the oat mixture.
7. Mix all the ingredients together and form into a patty ¾ inch thick.
8. Spray a baking sheet with nonstick cooking spray and place the patty on the sheet. Bake for 5 to 6 minutes per side or until golden brown.
9. Set on the English muffin and top with the tomato and yogurt.

NUTRITION INFORMATION:

216 calories, 13g protein, 41g carbs, 2g fat

Chilled Asian Noodle Salad

INGREDIENTS

2 teaspoons Bragg Liquid Aminos

1 teaspoon rice wine vinegar (or white wine vinegar)

⅛ teaspoon freshly grated ginger

¼ teaspoon toasted sesame oil

1 green onion (scallion), white part only, chopped

4 ounces cooked chicken, sliced

¼ cup thinly sliced cucumber

¼ cup thinly sliced carrot

¼ cup thinly sliced red bell pepper

2 ounces of soba noodles, cooked according to package directions and chilled

DIRECTIONS

1. Whisk the Bragg Liquid Aminos, vinegar, ginger, sesame oil, and green onion in a small bowl and set aside.

2. Combine the chicken, vegetables, and noodles in a bowl.

3. Drizzle the dressing on top and toss.

NUTRITION INFORMATION:

260 calories, 30g protein, 21g carbs, 6g fat

Roasted Vegetables with Orange Balsamic Glaze

INGREDIENTS

½ small zucchini, diced

½ cup diced red bell pepper

½ tomato, diced

3 asparagus spears, woody stems trimmed, cut into 1-inch slices

Olive oil spray

2 teaspoons balsamic vinegar

2 teaspoons freshly squeezed orange juice

1 tablespoon minced shallot

½ cup cooked quinoa

3 ounces cooked chicken, cubed

1 tablespoon chopped fresh parsley

DIRECTIONS

1. Preheat the oven to 400°F.
2. Toss the zucchini, bell pepper, tomato, and asparagus in a bowl and coat with olive oil spray. Spread evenly on a rimmed baking sheet.
3. Roast for 5 minutes, then turn with a spatula and roast for another 5 minutes.
4. Mix the balsamic, orange juice, and shallot in a small bowl and drizzle over the hot vegetables. Roast for 5 more minutes.
5. When the vegetables are tender, toss with the quinoa, chicken, and parsley.

NUTRITION INFORMATION:

295 calories, 27g protein, 37g carbs, 4g fat

Sweet Potato and Black Bean Burrito

INGREDIENTS

Olive oil spray

½ yellow onion, chopped

¼ teaspoon ground cumin

¼ teaspoon cinnamon

¼ teaspoon cayenne

¼ teaspoon dried oregano

½ cup cubed (½-inch dice) sweet potato, unpeeled

½ small tomato, diced

3 ounces cooked chicken, shredded

¼ cup low-sodium canned black beans, drained and rinsed

1 10-inch whole-wheat tortilla

DIRECTIONS

1. Spray a skillet with olive oil and heat over medium heat.
2. Add the onion and sauté for about 5 minutes, until soft.
3. Add the spices and yam. Cook, stirring occasionally, until the sweet potatoes are fork-tender, approximately 8–10 minutes.
4. Mix in the tomato, chicken, and black beans and heat through.
5. Spoon into the tortilla and wrap like a burrito.

NUTRITION INFORMATION:

396 calories, 29g protein, 61g carbs, 4.6g fat

DELICIOUS DINNERS

Dinner may be the easiest of all the Skinny Rules meals—or at least the simplest. Remember that, in general, the fewer carbs the better, and, if possible, you should eat this meal at least three hours before bedtime. This means protein, fiber, protein, fiber, and—did I say this already?—protein and fiber. Here are some tasty entrees that will provide loads of both. They will also make you happy.

Roasted Vegetables with Pesto Spaghetti Squash

INGREDIENTS

1 cup cooked spaghetti squash (see step 1)

1 small tomato, seeded and diced

½ cup chopped red bell pepper

½ cup chopped zucchini

1 garlic clove, minced

Olive oil spray

Pesto (page 185)

DIRECTIONS

1. To prepare the squash, cut it in half and spoon out the center and seeds. Place in a glass baking dish cut side down. Add ¼ inch of water. Cover loosely with plastic wrap. Microwave on high for 15 minutes.
2. Meanwhile, preheat the oven to 450°F.
3. When the squash is done, use a fork to pull the flesh from the skin. The squash will form thin strands like spaghetti. Set aside 1 cup and keep warm. Reserve the rest in an air-tight container in the refrigerator for another meal.
4. Toss the tomato, bell pepper, and zucchini with the garlic. Coat evenly with olive oil spray.
5. Place the vegetables in a roasting pan, cover with foil, and roast for 20 minutes.
6. Toss the spaghetti squash with pesto and top with roasted vegetables.

NUTRITION INFORMATION:

219 calories, 24g protein, 23 carbs, 6g fat

Orange-Glazed Chicken

INGREDIENTS

Olive oil spray

1 tablespoon freshly squeezed orange juice

2 teaspoons agave

½ teaspoon freshly grated ginger

5 ounces boneless, skinless chicken breast

DIRECTIONS

1. Preheat the broiler. Line a baking sheet with foil and spray with olive oil.
2. Whisk the juice, agave, and ginger together in small bowl.
3. Brush both sides of the chicken with the glaze.
4. Broil for 5 minutes on each side.

NUTRITION INFORMATION:

175 calories, 26g protein, 9g carbs, 3g fat

Glazed Beet and Fennel Salad with Chicken

INGREDIENTS

1 small beet
1 cup arugula
1 cup mixed greens
¼ fennel bulb, thinly sliced
4 ounces cooked chicken, cubed
2 tablespoons coarsely chopped toasted almonds
Balsamic Dressing (page 182)

DIRECTIONS

1. Preheat the oven to 400°F.
2. Pierce the beet with a fork and wrap in foil. Roast for 45 minutes. Remove from the oven and let cool in the foil.
3. Unwrap the beet and use a paper towel to rub off the peel. Cut in half and slice in half-moon shapes.
4. Pile the arugula and mixed greens on a plate and top with fennel, beet, chicken, and almonds. Toss with the dressing.

NUTRITION INFORMATION:

206 calories, 23g protein, 13g carbs, 7g fat

Rosemary Lemon Salmon with Roasted Asparagus

INGREDIENTS

6 large asparagus spears

Olive oil spray

freshly ground black pepper

4 ounces wild salmon, deboned

1 teaspoon freshly squeezed lemon juice

1 sprig of fresh rosemary

2 lemon slices

DIRECTIONS

1. Preheat the oven to 400°F. Cover a baking sheet with foil.
2. Cut the woody ends off the asparagus (about 1 inch from the bottom) and place the spears on the baking sheet. Coat with olive oil spray. Sprinkle a dash of black pepper over the asparagus and toss. Line up the spears in single layer.
3. Place the salmon on top of the asparagus. Drizzle with lemon juice. Place the rosemary sprig on the salmon and top with the lemon slices.
4. Roast for 12 to 15 minutes, until the salmon is flaky and the asparagus is deep green.

NUTRITION INFORMATION:

237 calories, 31g protein, 7g carbs, 9g fat

Steak Night with Cauliflower Mash and Spinach

INGREDIENTS

Olive oil spray

4 ounces loin steak (top sirloin, tenderloin, top loin), 1 inch thick

Freshly cracked black pepper

1½ cups chopped cauliflower

½ garlic clove

½ cup low-sodium vegetable broth

2 teaspoons grated parmesan cheese

¼ teaspoon dried thyme

2 cups fresh spinach

DIRECTIONS

1. Spray a medium-large skillet or wok with olive oil and heat over medium heat.
2. Season the steak with black pepper. Sear for at least 2 minutes on each side. Set aside to rest.
3. Place the cauliflower in a small pot with the broth and simmer, covered, for 5 to 7 minutes, until the cauliflower is fork-tender.
4. Transfer the cauliflower to a food processor, reserving the broth. Add the garlic and process until smooth, adding broth until the desired consistency is reached. Add parmesan and thyme and pulse to combine. It should be the thickness of mashed potatoes.
5. In a separate skillet, heat 2 tablespoons of the reserved cooking broth over medium heat. Add the spinach, cover, and cook over medium heat for 1 to 2 minutes, until the spinach is wilted.
6. Place the spinach and cauliflower on a plate alongside the steak.

NUTRITION INFORMATION:

341 calories, 27g protein, 10g carbs, 21g fat

Asian Salmon over Sesame Kale

INGREDIENTS

1 teaspoon Dijon mustard

1 teaspoon Bragg Liquid Aminos

¼ teaspoon grated fresh ginger

¼ teaspoon minced garlic

5 ounces wild salmon

2 cups chopped kale

1 teaspoon toasted sesame oil

DIRECTIONS

1. Preheat the oven to 400°F.
2. Mix the Dijon, Bragg Liquid Aminos, ginger, and garlic together in a small bowl.
3. Brush both sides of the salmon with the mixture.
4. Put fish in a baking dish, and bake for 10 to 12 minutes, until the fish flakes when probed with a fork.
5. Meanwhile, steam the kale for 2 minutes, just long enough to wilt it. Toss with sesame oil.
6. Place the salmon atop the wilted kale.

NUTRITION INFORMATION:

378 calories, 41g protein, 15g carbs, 9g fat

Seared Pork with Lemon-Thyme Sauce

This dish is very nice served alongside Roasted Tomatoes (page 177) and a salad.

INGREDIENTS

    Olive oil spray
    4 ounces thinly cut pork loin chop
    Freshly cracked black pepper
    ¼ cup low-sodium chicken or vegetable broth
    1 tablespoon freshly squeezed lemon juice
    1 teaspoon chopped fresh thyme
    ½ garlic clove, minced

DIRECTIONS

1. Heat a skillet over medium-high heat and lightly spray with olive oil.
2. Season the loin with cracked pepper. Place in the skillet and sear for 2 minutes on each side. Transfer to a plate and set aside.
3. Add the broth, lemon juice, thyme, and garlic to the skillet and heat over medium heat. Simmer until sauce reduces slightly, 2 to 3 minutes.
4. Add the pork to the sauce and cook until no longer pink, 2 to 3 more minutes.

NUTRITION INFORMATION:

    235 calories, 33.7g protein, 2g carbs, 9.5g fat

Feta and Basil–Stuffed Chicken Breast with Roasted Zucchini

INGREDIENTS

Olive oil spray

1 tablespoon crumbled feta cheese

1 tablespoon chopped fresh basil

1 tablespoon finely chopped sundried tomatoes

5 ounces boneless, skinless chicken breast, pounded to ½-inch thickness

1 medium zucchini, sliced into ¼-inch-thick rounds

Dash of freshly ground black pepper

DIRECTIONS

1. Preheat the oven to 350°F. Lightly spray a baking dish with olive oil.
2. In a small bowl, mix the feta, basil, and sundried tomatoes. Set aside.
3. Lay the chicken in the baking dish. Place the feta mixture in the center of the chicken. Fold the chicken over the filling and secure with toothpicks.
4. Add the zucchini rounds to the dish and spray lightly with olive oil. Season with black pepper.
5. Bake for 15 to 20 minutes, until the chicken is done (it's no longer pink and the juices run clear) and the zucchini is tender.

NUTRITION INFORMATION:

250 calories, 36g protein, 10g carbs, 2.6g fat

Cajun Tilapia Pocket

INGREDIENTS

Olive oil spray
6 ounces wild tilapia fillet
½ lime
1 teaspoon Cajun seasoning
4 asparagus spears, woody ends trimmed
½ medium red bell pepper, cut into thin strips
6 cherry tomatoes, halved
Freshly ground black pepper

DIRECTIONS

1. Preheat oven to 375°F. Lightly spray a large sheet of foil with olive oil.
2. Place the tilapia on the foil. Squeeze the lime half over both sides of the fillet, then pat with Cajun seasoning on both sides.
3. Spray the asparagus, bell pepper, and tomatoes with olive oil and toss with black pepper. Add the vegetables to the foil alongside the tilapia.
4. Fold the foil to form a pouch and crimp the ends. Place directly on the oven rack (or on a sheet pan if you're worried about the contents leaking out) and bake for 20 to 25 minutes, until the fish is cooked through, flaky on the inside, and the vegetables are tender.

NUTRITION INFORMATION:

214 calories, 37g protein, 11g carbs, 3.5g fat

Mediterranean Halibut with Arugula and Avocado Salad

INGREDIENTS

Olive oil spray

¼ teaspoon chopped fresh oregano

⅛ teaspoon chopped fresh thyme

1 tablespoon chopped kalamata olives

6 cherry tomatoes, quartered

2 teaspoons freshly squeezed lemon juice

5 ounces halibut fillet

2 cups arugula

¼ avocado, sliced

1 small tomato, sliced

Dash of freshly ground black pepper

DIRECTIONS

1. Preheat the oven to 375°F. Cover a baking sheet with foil, and then lightly spray the foil with olive oil.
2. In a small bowl, stir the oregano, thyme, olives, tomatoes, and lemon juice together.
3. Place the halibut on the foil and top with the olive-tomato mixture.
4. Place baking sheet in the oven and bake for 20 to 25 minutes, until the fish is flaky and cooked through.
5. Top the arugula with avocado, tomato, and pepper.
6. Serve the fish alongside the salad.

NUTRITION INFORMATION:

258 calories, 28g protein, 14g carbs, 11g fat

Italian Turkey Burger

INGREDIENTS

Olive oil spray

4 ounces ground white meat turkey

2 tablespoons canned crushed tomato

½ teaspoon dried Italian seasoning

⅛ teaspoon garlic powder

1 tablespoon grated parmesan cheese

DIRECTIONS

1. Heat a small skillet over medium-high heat. Coat with olive oil spray.
2. In a small bowl, combine all the remaining ingredients and mix well, using your hands. Form into a patty.
3. Place the patty in the skillet and sear for 4 minutes on each side or until no longer pink in the center.

NUTRITION INFORMATION:

198 calories, 25g protein, 4g carbs, 9.6g fat

Chicken Chopped Salad

INGREDIENTS

Herb-Roasted Chicken Breast (page 167)

2 cups chopped mixed greens

¼ cup chopped jarred roasted pepper

¼ cup chopped tomato

1 Persian cucumber, chopped

2 tablespoons low-sodium canned garbanzo beans, drained and
rinsed

1 tablespoon Mustard Vinaigrette (page 184)

DIRECTIONS

Cube the chicken and toss lightly with all ingredients.

NUTRITION INFORMATION:

271 calories, 28g protein, 18g carbs, 10.5g fat

Wild Salmon with Lemon Herb Oil and Roasted Tomatoes

INGREDIENTS

Olive oil spray

1 teaspoon freshly squeezed lemon juice

1 teaspoon olive oil

1 teaspoon chopped fresh oregano (or ½ teaspoon dried)

1 teaspoon chopped fresh basil

5 ounces wild salmon fillet

1 cup Roasted Tomatoes (page 177)

DIRECTIONS

1. Preheat the oven to 450°F. Spray a sheet of foil with olive oil.
2. Mix the lemon juice, olive oil, oregano, and basil together in a small bowl.
3. Put the fish on the foil and coat with the lemon-herb oil. Bake for 8 to 10 minutes, until the fish flakes when probed with a fork.
4. Serve with roasted tomatoes.

NUTRITION INFORMATION:

338 calories, 32g protein, 16g carbs, 12g fat

Salmon and Lime Cakes Over Sautéed Swiss Chard

INGREDIENTS

Olive oil spray

6 ounces skinless wild salmon fillet

1 teaspoon grated lime zest

1 teaspoon fresh ginger, finely minced

1 tablespoon chopped fresh parsley

1 large egg white

½ red bell pepper, chopped

⅛ red onion, thinly sliced

½ garlic clove, minced

2 cups chopped Swiss chard leaves, ribs removed

DIRECTIONS

1. Preheat the oven to 400°F. Line a baking sheet with foil and spray it with olive oil.

2. Cut the salmon into chunks.

3. Put the salmon, lime zest, ginger, parsley, egg white, and pepper in a food processor. Pulse until combined.

4. Shape into two patties with your hands and place on the baking sheet. Bake for 12 to 15 minutes, until the salmon is opaque in the center.

5. Meanwhile, heat a skillet over medium-high heat. Coat with olive oil spray. Add the onion and garlic and sauté for 5 minutes.

6. Add the Swiss chard and cook until just wilted.

7. Place the chard on a plate and top with the salmon cakes.

NUTRITION INFORMATION:

262 calories, 32g protein, 19g carbs, 7g fat

Parmesan-Crusted Chicken

INGREDIENTS

    1 tablespoon grated parmesan cheese

    Dash of freshly ground black pepper

    5 ounces boneless, skinless chicken breast

    ½ tablespoon Dijon mustard

DIRECTIONS

1. Preheat the oven to 400°F.
2. Combine the parmesan and pepper on a small plate.
3. Pat the chicken dry with a paper towel and lightly coat with mustard.
4. Dredge with the parmesan mixture until fully coated.
5. Place on a baking sheet and bake for 10 to 12 minutes, until no longer pink in the center. Serve with roasted vegetables or a side salad.

NUTRITION INFORMATION:

    157 calories, 29g protein, 0.2g carbs, 3g fat

Farmer's Market Greens with Chicken

INGREDIENTS

1 teaspoon Dijon mustard

1 tablespoon white balsamic vinegar

3 cups chopped mixed greens

6 ounces cooked boneless, skinless chicken breast, chopped

1 Persian cucumber, sliced thin

1 small tomato, seeded and sliced

½ carrot, unpeeled, sliced thin

DIRECTIONS

1. Combine the mustard and vinegar in a small bowl. Whisk together until smooth and set aside.

2. Combine all remaining ingredients in a salad bowl. Drizzle the dressing on top and toss.

NUTRITION INFORMATION:

228 calories, 35g protein, 10g carbs, 4g fat

Braised Halibut

- -

INGREDIENTS

Olive oil spray

2 tablespoons chopped leeks (white part only), thoroughly cleaned

½ teaspoon chopped fresh thyme

5 ounces halibut fillet

¼ cup low-sodium vegetable broth

DIRECTIONS

1. Heat a small skillet over medium-high heat and coat with olive oil spray.
2. Sauté the leeks for 4 minutes, or until soft.
3. Add the thyme and heat for 2 minutes, stirring. Set the fish on the leeks and sauté for 3 minutes on each side.
4. Add the broth and cook for another 3 minutes.

NUTRITION INFORMATION:

145 calories, 28g protein, 4g carbs, 3g fat

Pesto-Roasted Chicken Breast

INGREDIENTS

2 cups chopped assorted vegetables for roasting (eggplant, bell pepper, yellow squash, zucchini, tomato, etc.)

2 tablespoons Pesto (page 185)

5 ounces boneless, skinless chicken breast

DIRECTIONS

1. Preheat the oven to 400°F. Line a baking sheet with foil.
2. Toss the vegetables with 1 tablespoon of the pesto. Slather the chicken breast with the other tablespoon of pesto.
3. Lay the vegetables on the baking sheet in a single layer. Place the chicken on top and roast for 12 to 15 minutes, or until the chicken is no longer pink inside.

NUTRITION INFORMATION:

223 calories, 30g protein, 15g carbs, 2g fat

Beef Ka-Bobs

Makes 4 servings

INGREDIENTS
¼ teaspoon black pepper

1 teaspoon dried cumin

1 garlic clove, finely minced

¼ cup white wine vinegar

2 tablespoons extra virgin olive oil

2 red bell peppers, cut into 1-inch squares

2 yellow onions, cut into 1-inch squares

2 zucchini, cut into ½-inch rounds

1 pound sirloin, cut into 1-inch cubes

DIRECTIONS
1. If using wooden skewers, start by soaking them. They should be immersed fully in water for at least 1 hour.
2. In a small bowl, combine the black pepper, cumin, garlic, vinegar, and olive oil.
3. Thread the skewers, alternating vegetables and meat. Place in a baking dish.
4. Pour the marinade over the skewers and cover. Refrigerate for at least 1 hour.
5. When the skewers are almost done marinating, preheat the grill. Grill over high heat, turning occasionally to cook each side (about 8 minutes total).

NUTRITION INFORMATION PER SERVING:
357 calories, 36g protein, 5g carbs, 7g fat

Fish Ka-Bobs

Makes 4 servings

INGREDIENTS

  2 tablespoons freshly squeezed lemon juice

  ¼ cup chopped fresh basil

  ¼ cup chopped fresh parsley

  1 garlic clove, finely minced

  2 tablespoons extra virgin olive oil

  1 pound fish (I often use skinless wild salmon), cut into 1-inch
     cubes

  12 cherry tomatoes

  1 large zucchini, cut into ½-inch rounds (you should have 12 pieces)

DIRECTIONS

1. If using wooden skewers, start by soaking them. They should be immersed fully in water for at least 1 hour.

2. In a small bowl, combine the lemon juice, basil, parsley, garlic, and olive oil.

3. Thread the skewers, alternating fish and vegetables. Place in a baking dish.

4. Pour the marinade over the skewers and cover. Refrigerate for 30 minutes (and no longer than 1½ hours).

5. When the skewers are almost done marinating, preheat the grill. Grill over medium-high heat, turning occasionally to cook each side, for 6 to 8 minutes total.

NUTRITION INFORMATION PER SERVING:

274 calories, 26g protein, 9g carbs, 10g fat

Red Curry Chicken with Kale

INGREDIENTS
½ tablespoon red curry paste

4 ounces boneless, skinless chicken breast, cut into 1-inch cubes

½ cup "lite" coconut milk

½ cup coarsely chopped mango

2 cups chopped kale

DIRECTIONS
1. Set a small pot over medium heat. Add the curry paste and heat for 1 minute.
2. Toss in the chicken and stir into the curry paste. Sear for 3 minutes, stirring occasionally.
3. Add the coconut milk and mango. Bring to boil, then reduce the heat and simmer for 6 minutes.
4. Add the kale and cook until wilted.

NUTRITION INFORMATION:
363 calories, 34g protein, 26g carbs, 6g fat

NOTES

INTRODUCTION

"Our results show that isolated aerobic": A Thorogood et al., "Isolated aerobic exercise and weight loss: a systematic review and meta-analysis of randomized controlled trials," *American Journal of Medicine*, 2011 Aug; 124(8): 747–755.

Not tons, but when researchers at the Marshfield Clinic: JJ Vanwormer, "Self-weighing frequency is associated with weight gain prevention over 2 years among working adults," *International Journal of Behavioral Medicine*, 2011 July 6.

The most convincing of these comes from Harvard's: F Hu et al., "Changes in diet and lifestyle and long-term weight gain in women and men," *New England Journal of Medicine*, 2011 June 23; 364(25): 2392–2404.

THE SKINNY RULES

Rule 1
Recently a group of Israeli: G Dubnov-Raz et al., "Influence of water drinking on resting energy expenditure in overweight children," *International Journal of Obesity*, 2011 Oct; 35(10): 1295–1300. Epub 2011 Jul 12.

Rule 2
"First," they write, "humans may lack a physiological": BM Popkin et al., "A short history of beverages and how our body treats them," *Obesity Reviews*, 2008 Mar; 9(2): 151–155.

Rule 3
That is what a group of Icelandic: L Thorsdottir et al., "Randomized trial of weight-loss diets for young adults varying in fish and fish oil content," *International Journal of Obesity* (London), 2007 Oct; 31(10): 1560–1566.

His response? "So be a vegan who eats bacon!": R Lynch, "Chef Tal Ronnen's flavorful veganism," *Los Angeles Times*, June 23, 2011, E1.

Rule 4

Björck tried an experiment: I Björck, "A novel wheat variety with elevated content of amylose increases resistant starch formation and may beneficially influence glycaemia in healthy subjects," *Food and Nutrition Research.* Epub August 22, 2011, Vol. 55i0.70–74.

Rule 5

As reported in a recent nutrition journal: PR Newby et al., *"Intake of whole grains, refined grains, and cereal fiber measured with 7-day diet records and associations with risk factors for chronic disease,"* American Journal of Clinical Nutrition, 2007 December, 86(6): 1745–1753.

See also N Rose, ed. *Journal of Nutrition and Education Behavior,* 2007 March; 39(2): 90–94.

And the Baltimore Longitudinal Study of Aging reported: PK Newby, et al., "Intake of whole grains, refined grains, and cereal fiber measured with 7-day diet records and association with risk factors for chronic disease," *American Journal of Clinical Nutrition,* 2007 December, v 86. 1745–53.

Rule 6

"Overall, whole apple increased satiety more than": B Rolls et al., "The effect of fruit in different forms on energy intake and satiety at a meal," *Appetite,* 2009 April; 52(2): 416–422.

"A well-balanced diet can equally improve": F Magkos et al., "Organic food: nutritious food or food for thought? A review of the evidence," *International Journal of Food Science,* 2003 Sep; 54(5): 357–371.

Rule 8

Compared to people who didn't read labels: JN Variyam, "Do nutrition labels improve dietary outcomes?" *Health Economics,* 2008 June; 17(6): 695–708.

Another study, this one of more than 3,700: RE Post et al., "Use of nutrition facts label in chronic disease management: results from the National Health and Nutrition Examination Survey," *Journal American Dietetic Association,* 2010 April, 110(4):628–32.

Pro-technology Wired *magazine described polysorbate's:* Patrick Di Justo, "Cool Whip," Wired online, April 24, 2007, accessed January 12, 2012.

Also note: MSG is also used for making: World Health Organization, "Toxicological Evaluation of Certain Food Additives (prepared by the 31st meeting of JECFA)," 1988. WHO Food Additives Series No. 22, Cambridge University Press.

Rule 11

"For every additional daily serving of potatoes": F Hu et al., "Changes in diet and lifestyle and long-term weight gain in women and men," *New England Journal of Medicine,* 2011 June 23; 364(25): 2392–2404.

Each year, Americans consume more than 4.5: USDA Economic Research Service, "2008 Forecast," USDA ERS Reports, 2008.

Rule 12

No wonder Men's Health *magazine:* See http://www.menshealth.com/mhlists/ nutritious_foods_for_a_healthy_body/muscle_enhancer_lentils.php?page=2

One group ate 240 calories of pretzels: D Heber et al., "Pistachio nuts reduce triglycerides and body weight by comparison to refined carbohydrate snack in obese subjects on a 12-week weight loss program," *Journal of the American College of Nutrition,* 2010 June; 29(3): 198–203.

This led them to proclaim: RD Mattes et al., "Impact of peanuts and tree nuts on body weight and healthy weight loss in adults," *Journal of Nutrition,* 2008 Sep; 138(9): 1741S–1745S.

Rule 13

The connection is so strong that: B Morgenstern et al., "Fast food and neighborhood stroke risk," *Annals of Neurology,* 2009 Aug; 66(2): 165–170.

Rule 14

From the University of Massachusetts Medical School: M Yunsheng et al., "Association between eating patterns and obesity in a free-living US adult population," *American Journal of Epidemiology,* 2003 July 1; 158(1): 85–92.

From the journal Pediatrics: MT Timlin et al., "Breakfast eating and weight change in a 5-year prospective analysis of adolescents: Project EAT (Eating Among Teens)," *Pediatrics,* 2008 Mar; 121(3): e638-645.

From the European Journal of Neuroscience: AP Goldstone et al., "Fasting biases brain reward systems towards high-calorie foods," *European Journal of Neuroscience,* 2009 Oct; 30(8): 1625–1635.

Rule 15

When scholars writing in the journal Appetite: SH Fay et al., "What determines real-world meal size? Evidence for pre-meal planning," *Appetite,* 2011 April; 56(2): 284–299. Epub 2011 Jan 11.

Rule 17

That's why vegetable soup: B Rolls et al., "Serving large portions of vegetable soup at the start of a meal affected children's energy and vegetable intake," *Appetite,* 2011 Aug; 57(1): 213–219. Epub 2011 May.

Scientists at Johns Hopkins single out kale and broccoli: L Dinkova-Kostova et al., "Induction of the phase 2 response in mouse and human skin by sulforaphane-containing broccoli sprout extracts," *Cancer Epidemiology Biomarkers,* 2007 April; 16(4): 847–851.

Rule 19

Some experts estimate that 20 percent: M Ohayon et al., "Meta-analysis of quantitative sleep parameters from childhood to old age," *Sleep,* 2004 Nov 1; 27(7): 1255–1273.

"Alterations in the balance between sleep": AV Nedeltcheva et al., "Sleep curtailment is accompanied by increased intake of calories from snacks," *American Journal of Clinical Nutrition,* 2009 Jan; 89(1): 126–133.

THE SKINNY WAY

In 2009, the Brookhaven National Laboratory: GJ Wang et al., "Evidence of gender differences in the ability to inhibit brain activation elicited by food," *Proceedings of the National Academy of Sciences,* 2009 Jan 27; 106(4): 1249–1254.

ACKNOWLEDGMENTS

I have to say that this book was so much fun to write, thanks largely to my writing partner, Greg Critser. His sense of humor and passion for this book were a perfect match to my energy, and the plan came together seemingly effortlessly as we worked. Greg's nephew's anecdotes, shared on a weekly basis, were incredibly helpful.

Thanks to my right-hand "man," Nicole Trinler, for enduring my schedule and wrangling me in to work when I was completely exhausted and irritable! Nicole always stays consistent and keeps me on track. This book wouldn't have gotten done in time without her.

I want to thank my agents, Brett Hansen and Richard Abate, for their dedication to this book and focus on my career. I would not be where I am today without the help of Brett Hansen.

At the risk of sounding like an actor accepting an Oscar, I want to thank my lawyer, P.J. Shapiro. He makes sure everything gets signed, sealed, and delivered.

A big shout-out to Marnie Cochran, editor at Ballantine. I had a million meetings in New York shopping this book but when I met her, I knew immediately that she "got me." She was ready to go to work on this project that very day and I love that kind of person. I'm a big believer in hitting the ground running because that is how you make things happen, and Marnie operates that way, too.

Thanks also to the whole team at Ballantine and their tireless efforts on this project. I'm so happy to work with such a powerful and prestigious publishing house.

Thank you to my best friend, Justin Anderson. He tries to keep me sane in an insane business and, let me tell you, that is an almost impossible job. Justin is also one of the coolest people I know.

Thanks to my producer on *The Biggest Loser*, Joel Relampagos, for getting the best out of me at work. The person you see on my show is because of Joel. He is the best producer I have ever worked with.

Last but not least are a list of the closest people in my life that make me who I am: Cristi Conaway, Mark Murphy, Coco Murphy, Miles Murphy, Ally George (my Mee), Kate Angelo, Eric Duffy, Michael Martin, Darren Gold, and Pat Grantham. I love all of you very much.

Ah, but wait! I have one other being to acknowledge! Thank you, Karl—my wonderful dog! I was introduced to Karl almost two years ago. He had been abandoned and was near comatose with the pain of his many injuries. I immediately fell in love with him. From the beginning of our relationship, I have carried him everywhere. He is funny, charismatic, and above all else, so chill. While I worked on this book, he was right at my feet and as I'm writing this, he is in the chair beside me snoring. He reminds me about unconditional love and about trying not to sweat the bad stuff. I have learned a lot from that little mutt. . . . Okay, I gotta go squeeze him really hard right now.

INDEX

ABOUT THE AUTHORS

BOB HARPER is a world-renowned fitness trainer and star of the NBC reality series *The Biggest Loser,* which finished its thirteenth season in 2012. With several bestselling fitness DVDs, his own line of supplements, an online fitness club, as well as the inspirational book *Are You Ready!* to his credit, Harper still teaches a local spin class where he resides in Los Angeles, with his dog, Karl. For more information go to www.mytrainerbob.com.

GREG CRITSER is a longtime science and medical journalist. The author of the international bestseller *Fat Land: How Americans Became the Fattest People in the World,* he lives in Pasadena, California.

THE SKINNY RULES

RULE 1: Drink a Large Glass of Water Before Every Meal—No Excuses!

RULE 2: Don't Drink Your Calories

RULE 3: Eat Protein at Every Meal—or Stay Hungry and Grouchy

RULE 4: Slash Your Intake of Refined Flours and Grains

RULE 5: Eat 30 to 50 Grams of Fiber a Day

RULE 6: Eat Apples and Berries Every Single Day. Every. Single. Day!

RULE 7: No Carbs After Lunch

RULE 8: Learn to Read Food Labels So You Know What You Are Eating

RULE 9: Stop Guessing About Portion Size and Get It Right— for Good

RULE 10: No More Added Sweeteners, Including Artificial Ones

RULE 11: Get Rid of Those White Potatoes

RULE 12: Make One Day a Week Meatless

RULE 13: Get Rid of Fast Foods and Fried Foods

RULE 14: Eat a Real Breakfast

RULE 15: Make Your Own Food and Eat at Least Ten Meals a Week at Home

RULE 16: Banish High-Salt Foods

RULE 17: Eat Your Vegetables—Just Do It!

RULE 18: Go to Bed Hungry

RULE 19: Sleep Right

RULE 20: Plan One Splurge Meal a Week

(cut this page out and post where you'll see it daily)